Praise for *Baby Rollercoaster: Secret Sorrow of Infe*

AMAZING! Janice Colven's writing flows with such ease and is so relatable. I wish so much that I had been able to read this while I was at the beginning of my struggle. This book is an emotional guide for those going through infertility or those that are willing to take the time to understand those that are. I learned – that I am not alone! That there is so much purpose beyond children. That two is a family!

~Jillian Smith

This book is written from the heart of someone who has traveled a long emotional journey through infertility. This book is perfect for anyone on this journey who is looking for answers to questions or assurance that what they are going through someone else has experienced. Although their journey may not be exactly the same, they may be able to draw on some of the experiences and know they are not alone in what they are feeling. I was surprised by the emotional impact this book had on me. I found myself holding my breath (even though I didn't realize it) and often tearing up at the various steps along the journey. The book drew me and held my attention to the end. I would recommend this book to anyone who is following the path of infertility and is searching for answers along the way.

~JoAnne Sigurdson

10/10 recommend! I couldn't seem to put this book down! I loved how the author included deep and dark moments but also threw things in that made me laugh! The author wrote that she experienced a rollercoaster of emotions throughout her journey, but as a reader, I did too! I laughed, cried, and got goosebumps!

Baby Rollercoaster is the PERFECT title – this book will take you on a "rollercoaster" of emotions as you connect with a woman who has experienced infertility and the emotions of sorrow and hope it brought her. This book would be perfect for women that are experiencing infertility or people who are close to those who have or are experiencing infertility (such as a sister or daughter). I was surprised by the amount of money and pain (both emotionally and physically) IVF is. I learned straight-up facts about infertility which I think is important for readers to know.

~Ellen Krogan

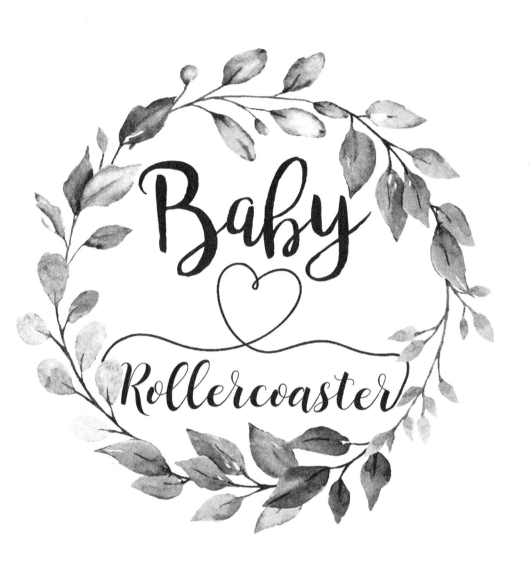

Baby ♡ Rollercoaster

THE UNSPOKEN SECRET SORROW OF INFERTILITY

JANICE COLVEN

Baby Rollercoaster – The Unspoken Secret Sorrow of Infertility
Copyright 2021 Janice Colven

Published by:
Wood Dragon Books
Post Office Box 429
Mossbank, Saskatchewan, Canada S0H3G0

ISBN: 978-1-989078-58-7

Contact the author regarding speaking to your group at babyrollercoaster@outlook.com

Follow the author on Instagram @janice_colven

Find her book on Facebook at Baby Rollercoaster – A book by Janice Colven

For every woman
who knows the unspoken secret sorrow
of infertility.

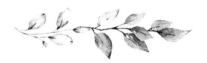

"There is a unique pain that comes from preparing a place in your heart for a child that never comes."

- David Platt

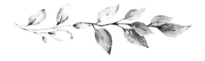

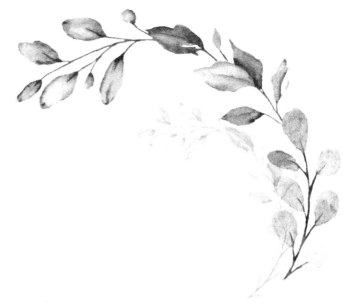

Introduction

From the time I was a little girl, I dreamed of being a mom. I took for granted that motherhood would be in my future.

I had a loving and nurturing spirit from an early age. I loved baby dolls and everything that went with them. My favorite baby was Gail. I named her after my dance teacher, who I adored. I brought Gail everywhere.

She was a "newborn" baby doll. She looked like an infant with a bald head and painted on eyes. She came with real diapers and a baby bottle filled with a white liquid that looked like milk. When I turned the bottle upside down to feed Gail, the milk seemed to vanish, as if my baby doll was actually drinking the milk. Feeding and caring for my doll felt so real.

I took great pleasure and responsibility in nurturing Gail. I imitated the things my mom did for my little brother—like rocking, feeding, and changing diapers. I loved her sleepers and bibs and changed her outfits often. Gail slept in a little pink crib, complete with a frilly canopy, next to my bed—which was also pink and frilly. I fell asleep each night content that my baby was sleeping, safe and sound beside me.

My heart and imagination may have been in the right place, but I had a lot to learn about being a mother.

One day, my family went to the city to shop at Woolco—a bargain hunter's paradise that was eventually acquired by Walmart. Naturally, I had Gail with me. I dutifully carried her through Woolco while my mom shopped. I loved searching through the aisles and bins and playing with Gail among the store racks while Mom browsed. Eventually, I must've grown weary of my motherly responsibilities because when we arrived at the checkout, I tenderly placed Gail up onto the counter and proceeded to admire the nearby candy shelves. The clerk was horrified when Gail rolled along the conveyor belt with our purchases. She thought my doll was a real baby! To my five-year-old self, Gail was a real baby. I loved her with all my heart, even if she did get heavy after I had carried her around for an afternoon of shopping.

Gail briefly took second place in my affections when Christmas morning arrived the year I was six. Santa brought me a baby doll that ate and wet herself. She came with special packets of powdered food in wildly delicious flavors like strawberry, banana, and peas. When the powdered packets were mixed with water in the special dish that came with the doll, a brightly colored paste appeared. Once the "food" was mixed and ready, I pressed a button on my doll's back and magically, she came to life.

Her mouth produced a mechanical sound that was followed by a rhythmic opening and closing of her mouth which simulated a chewing motion. I was elated. I finally had the baby of my dreams. I dutifully spooned the sticky, gooey, mess into the doll's mouth. The food flowed through her hard, plastic body and out into her diaper which I quickly changed into a fresh diaper, just like I had watched my mom do for my little brother many times. I was in love with this new baby doll. Even though I was only six years old, my mothering instincts were already in full force.

I spent countless hours with my doll—mixing her special food, feeding her, and changing her diaper. This amazing doll brought me so much pleasure and pride in my ability to care for her. In my six-year-old eyes, she was perfect. My mom thought so, too, except that the constant mixing, feeding, and diaper changing process was messy, the brightly colored food stained everything it touched, and we already had a real baby—my little brother—that ate and needed diaper changes. I quickly learned that this baby doll could not eat Christmas cookies or other bits and bites from my plate. The special food and tiny diapers that had come with the doll quickly ran out and the novelty wore off. Gail was still my favorite doll.

My love extended to babies that did not come from a box or a store. One day, when I was seven years old, I found a dead gopher in front of our house. I wrapped it up in a soft, pink blanket and gently placed the gopher in Gail's stroller. I meandered down the lane in the bright summer sun with my newfound baby wrapped up tight. I figured I could coax the gopher back to health and we'd have a great time then.

Unfortunately, my afternoon ended with a hot bath, the lingering scent of Ivory soap, and a scolding from my mom about dead things and fleas. I was grief-stricken to learn that death was final and no amount of love could bring that gopher back to life. Mom wisely convinced me to reinstate Gail back to her rightful place in her freshly sanitized stroller and to leave the gophers alone—dead or alive.

Eventually, baby dolls lost their appeal. I wanted a real baby. I looked around and saw—my little brother. He was perfect! Blond-haired and blue-eyed, he looked adorable in a lacy dress and pink lipstick. Though when I tried to style his hair, he finally rebelled. He simply wouldn't hold still for curls. My brother was most definitely a boy and planned to keep playing in the dirt and running wild in the golden wheat fields around our house. Curlers and hairspray didn't fit into his definition of himself as a boy. After my brother's rejection of the role of real baby, I had to go back to playing with Gail once again.

When I was eight, my mom announced that she was going to have a baby. I was elated! I had dreamed my whole life of having a little sister and immediately set my heart on the baby being a girl.

I waited impatiently during the course of my mom's pregnancy. I was anxious to know if the baby was a boy or a girl. My mom had a difficult pregnancy and spent four weeks before delivery in the hospital. My brother and I stayed at home with Dad and Grandma. When the day finally came that Mom was scheduled to deliver our new baby, Dad drove us to the city, a three-hour drive from our farm in southern Saskatchewan. We stayed in a hotel. It had a pool. Dad took us swimming and fed us McDonald's and let us stay up way too late watching cartoons and eating snacks from the vending machine in the lobby.

The next morning dawned dark, cold, and blustery—a typical February morning on the prairies. We piled into our little car and drove through the early morning city traffic to the hospital. Grandma had come along to watch my brother and me while Dad went with Mom to the delivery room. I remember a really long wait in a really long hallway on the maternity ward. My brother kept having to go to the bathroom or needing a snack from the cafeteria—as four-year-olds do—and every time we left the waiting area, I was upset. I was worried we were going to miss seeing our baby. I could barely stand the suspense.

Finally, the doors at the end of the hall opened and a nurse appeared, pushing a bassinette. I will remember the little bassinette coming down the hallway for the rest of my life. It was pink! The nurse stopped and I caught my first glimpse of that beautiful baby girl—my sister.

We named her Rhonda.

My mom worked long hours helping my dad on the farm and teaching at the community college in our small town. I often took care of my sister while Mom was busy. I knew how to comfort her when she cried and how to make her laugh and coo. I knew her favorite snacks and how to prepare them. I read her stories and played with her. I loved her completely.

As Rhonda grew older, I extended my sisterly duties to include things like guiding her fashion choices and hairstyles. When Rhonda was four, her favorite outfit was a black bodysuit with a Mickey Mouse figure printed on the front. It was a hand-me-down I had worn with a tutu for a dance recital a few years earlier. My sister loved that bodysuit and wore it every day for weeks even though I—with my superior twelve-year-old fashion sense—tried to convince her to change into something else. I didn't know it then, but these experiences—from caring for Rhonda when she was a baby to guiding her fashion sense as she grew older—would be the beginning of an unbreakable bond.

This bond grew from unconditional love, and eventually friendship, as we matured into adulthood. Our connection strengthened as we each started hitting the milestones that make up life. Graduations, new jobs, falling in love, and marrying were leaps of faith that we celebrated together. After we were both married, we waited for the eventual next step in our adult lives—motherhood.

For some, the road to motherhood is a straightforward, traditional trajectory. Grow up, fall in love, get married, have children. For other women, the road to motherhood is a rollercoaster of emotions and a far less traditional ride.

In both cases, women start off with similar expectations of what motherhood will look like, what the timeline will be, and what we will do when we get there. We buy the map to motherhood and have the trip planned down to the smallest detail. We dream of the day that we will cuddle our own bundle of joy. We imagine the nursery, the first birthday party, the fresh and powdery smell of our newborn. We feel that deep sense of love and longing to care for our child instinctively. We are born with motherhood in our hearts.

Not only are we born with motherhood hardwired, but we purchase our tickets and hop into what we anticipate will be a slow and steady merry-go-round ride. Our moms buy us baby dolls and show us how to take care of them. Our families praise our nurturing spirit and shape us to express motherly traits. As young girls, we care for our siblings and babysit during our teenage years. All the while, training for motherhood.

But what happens when you've planned the trip, you're at the fair, and you find yourself on a rollercoaster instead of a merry-go-round? You ascend to the top of the track and quickly realize that you're about to take a sharp twist and then there's an unexpected turn followed by a terrifying drop and you're not ready for any of it. It's in this moment that you're hit with the fact that you're aboard the *Drop of Doom* coaster when really, you thought you purchased a ticket for a much less extreme ride. You catch glimpses of couples on the other rides—the gentle ones, the predictable ones. You can hear their laughter and you see them smiling and holding hands in the warm sunshine. It's a stark contrast to the screams you hear and white knuckles you see on your rollercoaster ride.

At first, you're resilient and bounce back after the adrenaline of the sudden drop subsides. You hope with each rise that the next turn will be gentler and that the next twist will take you to the gate. You want off that rollercoaster, but you're there, strapped in tight, for the whole ride. You can't get off and there's no escape route. You feel powerless and begin to lose hope.

Soon, your natural reserve of resilience depletes and your tolerance to the uncertainty of each unwelcome twist or turn, diminishes. It takes you longer to recover when your coaster car crashes down from the top of the track at breakneck speed and slams into the lowest of lows. You lose sight of why you even boarded the rollercoaster in the first place. You stop being able to imagine your arrival at the exit, that the ride will ever end. Time whizzes by in a blur of colors and sounds. You try, but you can't take it in or enjoy it. You need every ounce of strength to hold on and to keep your seat on the ride. You turn and look to your husband. His expression mirrors the fearful and defeated look that is etched on your own face. The ride is hell. He wants off as badly as you do.

Your family and friends watch from the ground as you and your partner brace yourselves for the plummets. They're powerless to help you and shout words that are meant to encourage, but fall far short of comfort. This ride wasn't what you dreamed it would be. Your heart and your stomach can't take any more. You need to get off.

Experiencing infertility is much like riding that emotional rollercoaster. It's a cycle of hope, devastation, sadness, and grief on repeat. Infertility often comes up unexpectedly and blindsides us, flying in the face of the ingrained narrative that women should be mothers. This narrative shapes us to believe that motherhood is the only way we will find purpose in our lives or to fulfill our capacity to feel true love. That same archaic thinking pressures a woman to believe she is obligated and expected to bear a child to carry on a family name or a family business.

When a woman is walking through infertility, these all-too-common societal beliefs can impact her sense of value and purpose. The expectation of motherhood is perpetuated and reinforced with every sentimental country song about the joys of seeing two pink lines and every emotionally charged diaper commercial that touts the wonders of holding a newborn baby. As we age, the images of women as mothers change to depict us as grandmothers—arms wide open in a sunshiny meadow, waiting to embrace our adoring grandchildren. These are the narratives running through a woman's head as she quietly bears the unspoken secret sorrow of infertility.

This book is about my journey and my own personal baby rollercoaster ride. I wrote my story for the women who are walking the same infertility path. My story is also meant to provide insight for the women in our lives who love and support us through infertility. I want this book to inform you, to encourage you, and to inspire you to hope.

The story that you will read in the following pages is based on the events of my life. While some of the characters and details are fictitious, they are based on the very real moments and raw emotions that I experienced over the course of my infertility and my life after infertility.

I want you to know that this path is not easy, that there are some dark times along the way—but that even though it doesn't feel like life will ever be all right again, it will be. So, don't give up, hang on, be brave. You can be blessed with a great life and a happy life, even if it is not the life you had imagined.

Chapter 1

I am a teacher. One of my first teaching jobs was in a one-horse town—or one-tumbleweed town—surrounded by the patchwork fields and pumping oil wells of the Canadian prairies.

Imagine a bright-eyed and eager twenty-four-year-old girl fresh from the city, dressed in a skirt and heels, pulling up in front of a small, Kindergarten to Grade 12 school in a remote farming community, for a job interview. A tumbleweed slowly rolls down the road before her unbelieving eyes. I thought tumbleweeds only rolled down streets in western movies just before the bad guys rode into town on their horses, guns blazing. That was one of those moments when, looking back, I wonder, *what I was thinking*.

Tumbleweed or not, I went inside for the interview and was offered a teaching position on the spot. I asked for a day to consider the offer. Part of me wanted to shout "Yes!" and take the job immediately. Another part of me wasn't so sure. It was a tiny town, far from anywhere. The accommodations were dismal and there were few people my age for miles around. I wondered how I would make any friends—or worse—find a boyfriend. But, a small voice in my heart whispered, "Take it," and so, I did. Accepting the position would be a defining moment in my life. In this little town,

I would find my best friend and the love of my life. This little town was exactly where I needed to be.

I was young and enthusiastic, and I couldn't wait for the school year to begin. I spent countless hours in my new classroom preparing for my students, long before they were due to arrive. A kind-hearted soul was hard at work along with me. While I was decorating my back-to-school bulletin boards and writing lesson plans, she was making sure the school shined and smelled like fresh wax and lemon cleaner. Darlene was warm and friendly, and I liked her instantly.

We chatted often that first week. I must have made a good impression because the following week, Darlene said those infamous words every single girl loves to hear, "You just *have* to meet my son!"

Usually, when someone says this sort of thing, the natural response is, "Oh, sure! I would *love* to meet your son. Yes, I'm sure he's quite a nice guy." Nothing further is generally required, and usually, nothing more happens.

Darlene wasn't so easily deterred. Many conversations over the following months would include how I just *had* to meet her son. After talking with Darlene, I would sometimes find myself sitting at my desk, lesson plan half written, daydreaming about who this man, that I just *had* to meet, might be.

One afternoon in May, after almost a full year of not-so-subtle matchmaking, Darlene stopped by my house and invited me to a barbeque that evening. Our little town was deep in the heart of oil country and her son, Hoyt, the driller on a rig, was working close to town. Hoyt was staying with Darlene while he worked nearby as it saved him a night spent in a motel eating take out. According to Darlene, it would also be the perfect chance for me to meet him. I reluctantly agreed and then began agonizing over what to wear and what I would talk about once I arrived.

I primped, preened, and dressed, then walked to Darlene's house, where she invited me inside and introduced me to her son. I learned that Hoyt lived on a ranch only one hour from where I had grown up. He travelled across western Canada, working on drilling rigs in the oil field. He had worked his way up through the ranks and had recently accepted a promotion to the position of driller. I was instantly impressed by his hardworking spirit and the fact that he seamlessly managed a ranch while also leading a rig crew and working away from home for weeks at a time.

Hoyt had just arrived home after a long day spent on his drilling rig. He was still dressed in his safety boots and he had a smear of grease on his cheek. I'll never forget the moment we first met. He was tall with jade green eyes, blond hair, and golden-brown skin. For me—it was love at first sight.

Darlene's cat, Tigger, had greeted me when I entered the house, rubbing against my leg, purring, the way cats do. I was so nervous I started talking about what a great cat Tigger was, even though I am not a cat person. That night, I walked home with the stars bright above me and the sound of frogs croaking in the chilly spring air. I had a feeling that this meeting was just the beginning for Hoyt and me.

The next day at school, I asked Darlene to give my phone number to Hoyt. Just like that, it happened. All it took was one backyard barbeque and a mother's intuition. In that tiny town, I had found the love of my life. Soon, Hoyt and I were inseparable.

When Christmas arrived, we had been dating for six months. It seemed like the perfect time to meet Hoyt's extended family. My family is small, quiet, and conservative. Hoyt's family is large, rowdy, and fun. I was feeling a bit like a fish out of water at Hoyt's family Christmas celebration—plus I was the new girlfriend and was trying to make a good impression on all the aunties and cousins.

Picture thirty people, babies and kids happily playing, one large Christmas tree decorated with vintage ornaments, all crammed into a little farmhouse. The food was plentiful and traditional for this Ukrainian family—sour cabbage rolls, homemade perogies, turkey, and all the fixings. After a delicious meal, the women cleared the food and washed the dishes while the men visited around the kitchen table and the children played with their new toys. As the evening wore on, Hoyt's Grandpa brought out a bottle of whisky and insisted that we join him for a cup of Christmas cheer.

You should probably know I am a cheap drunk. After a few sips of whisky, I'll tell you all my secrets. What I didn't realize was what a "two-finger" drink was and how big Hoyt's Grandpa's fingers were. You should also know I have trouble saying no if it means hurting someone's feelings. So, when Grandpa poured me a drink and insisted I take it, I did. I thought the best way to handle this situation was to gulp the liquor down, finish it quickly, and be polite. I underestimated what a generous host Grandpa was. As soon as my glass was empty, he insisted on giving me a refill of the potent, amber-colored malt. He was likely thinking, "Hmm, this girl likes whisky, she'll fit in just fine!" So, I sat down with my full glass and sipped—slowly this time!

Soon the whisky started to work its magic, and my normally quiet and reserved personality gave way to reveal a much more outgoing side. Remember those secrets I mentioned earlier? Oh yes, I told them all. I proudly announced to a table full of people that I planned to have five (yes, that's right, five) little boys—and as soon as possible. *Yikes! What was I thinking?* We weren't even engaged yet and I was planning for five children. Luckily for me, Hoyt's family laughed and teased, but for some reason figured I was a keeper.

Soon after baring my soul to thirty almost-strangers, I started to feel whisky-induced tingling in my fingers and nose. It was time to go. I wasn't living with Hoyt yet, but his house was beginning to feel like home. When we were together, Hoyt and I spent hours, deep in conversation about our future. I started to keep a few of my belongings at his house and began to add my own personal touch to his home—a candle here and a photo frame there. Hoyt's house was quickly becoming our home. We knew with conviction that our forever was just beginning and had welcomed a puppy into our lives—it felt like the logical first step in our commitment together. We knew that this puppy was just the precursor to the children that would soon fill our home.

Riley, our new puppy, welcomed a surprise guest to his dog house in the barn that Christmas Eve. In my rosy glow, I insisted that I needed to play with Riley even though it was late at night and bitterly cold. After a few minutes of fetch and belly rubs, I grew tired and wanted to curl up with my wide-eyed puppy and sleep. Hoyt picked me up, dusted off the straw, took me from the cold floor of the barn to the warmth of his house, and put me to bed. I didn't know it at the time, but Hoyt would continue picking me up and dusting me off many more times on our journey to find our five little Colven boys. I learned that night always to pour my own drinks at Grandpa's house unless of course, I wanted to sleep with the dog.

Embarrassed, I called Darlene the next morning to apologize for my whisky-induced confessions. She laughed and said five grandsons would be just fine with her, but she warned me that five little boys could potentially be a handful. Just imagine the grass stains, the muddy boots, the hidden frogs, the flying hockey pucks, and the constant phone calls from the school.

"It won't be easy raising five boys," she said, "Raising Hoyt and his brother was sometimes challenging, but worth every moment. I can imagine your sons will be similar." I agreed wholeheartedly, and we hung up to go about our day, both of us anticipating the arrival of these little boys.

Hoyt and I knew shortly after meeting that his matchmaking mother had been right. We were meant to spend our lives together. We were married at Christmastime, almost one year to the day of my announcement at Christmas dinner. Like most young couples in love, we dreamed of having children and all the things we would do with our kids. We considered how much trouble a couple of Colven boys could cause together, and how we would parent our kids (I would be the bad cop, Hoyt would be the softie).

We enjoyed our first Christmas together as husband and wife, but we didn't go on an official honeymoon. Hoyt was due back to work on January 2. His rig was working in northern Alberta drilling oil wells in a remote, fly-in location. Hoyt was the driller on the rig crew—a leadership position—and he was needed to run the rig and lead the crew of men under his direction. Hoyt would be staying in a camp and would be away from home for a minimum of two weeks at a time, usually longer. Hoyt's dad, Doug, would make sure that our chores were done, the cows were healthy and cared for, and the snow was cleared in our yard so I could drive to work. Doug's help made it possible for Hoyt to be away from home.

We spent the days after Christmas preparing for Hoyt's departure—packing his warmest clothing, doing extra chores to relieve his dad of additional work, and soaking in every moment with each other. We knew those weeks apart would be long and lonely.

I went back to work, teaching Kindergarten, soon after the New Year. I was employed half-time that particular year which meant that after an hour-long commute from our farm, I spent my mornings singing, creating, and learning with twenty-five energetic children. I left the school at noon each day, covered in glue and sparkles, with a full heart. Being with my students lit up my soul—their laughter and energy were contagious. I felt fulfilled knowing that I was providing a classroom environment where these children could come to feel safe, connected, and valued each day—ideals that were not always a reality in their homes. I was able to make my students' days just a little bit brighter, safer, and happier. The fact that I could teach them as well, was a bonus. My nurturing spirit and mothering instinct were strong—even though I knew these students were not my own children.

Some afternoons, I was called to be a substitute teacher for the second half of my day. Other days, I went home and prepared lesson plans, cleaned my house, or checked on the cows for Hoyt. I spent the long winter evenings during those two week stretches that Hoyt was away, dreaming about our future. My vision always centered on a house full of children. It wouldn't occur to me for many years that this might not be the reality I would share with my husband.

Chapter 2

Our baby making began in earnest the summer after we were married. It was time; we were ready. The first six months of trying for our baby were exciting and full of anticipation. I was certain that I would soon be pregnant. I shared the news that we were trying for a baby with my mom who was overjoyed. Mom insisted that I choose a pattern and fabric so that she could begin quilting the blanket that would soon swaddle my newborn baby. I eagerly searched through countless bolts of pastel-colored fabric at a quilting shop to find the perfect material for a baby blanket. Picture a blue and coral theme. It would be suitable for a boy or a girl and it would match the soft grey color I would soon paint the nursery walls.

When my pregnancy test was negative month after month, "We'll try again" became our mantra. Eventually, our sense of anticipation started to turn into an awareness that something didn't feel right.

But what could possibly be the problem? We were both young and healthy and we knew about the birds and the bees. We searched "how to conceive" on Google and decided it was a straightforward process.

After one year of spinach eating, laying with my legs in the air, ovulation tracking, and college-level trying, we had no babies. No pregnancy symptoms. No positive tests. I had the uncomfortable feeling in the pit of my stomach that something was awry. It was time to go to the doctor. Something was wrong.

My first appointment was oddly comforting and unnerving at the same time. I had moved often since leaving home and my childhood doctor and I didn't have a family physician yet. I called several different offices until I found a doctor who was accepting new patients—a rarity in my town. I quickly learned there was a reason this particular doctor was accepting new patients. He likely had appointments available because the rest of the community knew what I did not—this particular doctor specialized in treating the elderly with their arthritis and high blood pressure, and steered clear of anything more complicated. He was certainly no authority on infertility. But he had an opening, so I went. I quickly came to realize why he was taking new patients when no other doctor for miles around had a moment in their schedule to spare.

The doctor arrived at the cramped and stuffy exam room late— shirt half tucked, glasses askew, and bushy mustache twitching. He called me "honey" and "dear" which should have been my first clue that he was not the doctor for me. Unfortunately, my manners kept me there with the faded abstract prints and ripped vinyl chairs from 1970. I explained the problem and waited for the cure.

He told me, "Have more sex! Don't watch TV or read in bed, stop playing hard-to-get! You're probably just missing your fertile window."

He was insinuating that I needed to initiate sex more often. He was suggesting that my negative pregnancy tests were my fault because my timing was off. I was embarrassed. Guilt and shame settled over me like a prickly, hot blanket.

I sat dumbfounded and unsure of how to respond.

The reality was, Hoyt and I were having sex every day. Ovulation predictor tests, cervical mucus tracking, and temperature charts were all in play to give us the precision and timing we hoped would result in pregnancy. Logically, if we had sex every day, we couldn't miss our opportunity for egg and sperm to meet.

Sex also caused me anxiety because with each cycle came the expectation that I would be pregnant. Each month, I'd stand expectantly over the sink in my bathroom, waiting and hoping that a second line would appear on the stick in my hand. But, no matter how hard I squinted or waved the pregnancy test in the air, it was always, devastatingly negative.

As I tried to take in this "advice," Dr. Mustache ended the appointment by peering knowingly over his glasses and reassuring me with these words, "Relax, and it will happen. Women are so impatient when they want to have a baby! Go home. You're young and there's nothing wrong with you. Be patient."

"What about my pain?!" I asked, bewildered. "I have extreme pain during my period. I can't sleep or stand for any amount of time. The pain lasts even after my period. I have pain during sex and if I use the bathroom. It shoots down my left leg and wraps around my back." I explained.

Dr. Mustache listened half-heartedly as he made notes in my chart. "You can take Advil if you have pain. Sometimes a warm heating pad helps, too."

His suggestions left me speechless.

That was the best medical advice this doctor had for me. I wish I had marched my twenty-seven-year-old self out of there and found a doctor I trusted, one who would listen to me, but instead, I went home and did as prescribed because he was the expert.

Dr. Mustache's nonchalant words that afternoon made me second-guess my intuition. His dismissiveness over my concerns and physical pain made me feel silly and reactionary. Although he may have eased some of my anxiety that something was wrong with my body, my fear that I was inadequate, or that I was doing something wrong, or that I was not trying hard enough to conceive—increased exponentially.

For six more months, I dutifully and anxiously followed Dr. Mustache's advice. I researched the topic of conception. I continued to track my cervical mucus and temperature. I timed my ovulation. I tolerated the pain in my lower left abdomen, even when I was doubled over and screaming, even when I was throwing up and the room was spinning, even when I couldn't sleep at night because the pain was too intense, even when handfuls of Advil didn't bring any relief—I kept going. I kept going because this was "normal" and I was just being impatient. I kept going even when Hoyt begged me to go back to Dr. Mustache or to get a second opinion.

I wanted to believe that I was healthy and that I could conceive a child. But my intuition disagreed, and as much as I tried to push down my fear, it kept popping back up like a beach ball that won't stay under the water.

Six months later, still, no baby.

I made another appointment to see Dr. Mustache. I explained that I was still concerned that something was wrong—I was still in incredible pain and I wasn't yet pregnant.

"If it'll make you feel better, let's get an ultrasound and some blood work done." He said as he peered over his glasses at me. Dr. Mustache's patronizing tone and insinuation that my pain was all in my head most certainly did not make me feel better—it infuriated me.

Dr. Mustache quickly scribbled something into my chart and checked boxes off of a requisition form. I left the exam room feeling like I had won a small victory and would hopefully soon have answers to my pain and infertility.

One week later, I arrived at the regional hospital where Dr. Mustache had referred me for an ultrasound and bloodwork. I checked in at the admitting desk, found a seat near the back of the reception area, and settled down to wait. When my name was called and it was my turn, I changed into a paper robe and entered the dimly lit ultrasound room. I shimmied onto the bed in my paper robe as elegantly as I could. With my feet in the stirrups, I waited for the ultrasound tech to begin the procedure.

Time stood still.

"Have you been experiencing pain during your cycle?" she asked.

Alarmed by the question, I quickly responded, "Yes, I have pain every month. It never stops. It starts in my lower left abdomen and wraps around my back and shoots down my left thigh. Using the bathroom hurts. Sex is painful. I can't find relief from the pain no matter how much Advil I take. It's awful." She continued to look at the blurry black screen and to make small notations on my chart.

"What do you see?" I anxiously asked.

Her reply did nothing to quell my growing fear. "You'll have to wait for the results. Your doctor will contact you in a few weeks."

I left the hospital that day with a mounting sense of foreboding deep in my soul. If only I could have known how a few simple tests would change the path my life was taking.

In a mental fog, I drove home and began the long wait for my results. Fourteen days later, I answered the call that my results were in and I could come in for an appointment with Dr. Mustache. I once again found myself sitting in a ripped vinyl chair, in that suffocating exam room, waiting to receive my fate.

Dr. Mustache entered the room and set my chart on the desk. I took a deep breath. This was it.

He said, "Well, we have the results of your ultrasound, my dear. There are two large tumors in your uterus. That is probably why you haven't conceived and possibly also why you're experiencing pain. But, we believe them to be benign."

My heart stopped and my breath caught in my chest. My throat started to close around the huge lump that always appears moments before my tears start to flow.

My first panicked question for Dr. Mustache was, "Can I still have a baby?" More questions started to come, faster and faster. "Will you remove the tumors? What caused them to form? How do you know they are benign? What if they aren't benign? If they are removed, how long will recovery take?"

My doctor put his hand on my arm, passed me a tissue, and said "Honey, I really can't comment on these things. You'll have to ask the gynecologist."

Exasperated with the lack of information and answers to my questions, I asked, "When can I go?"

Dr. Mustache's infuriating response was that it would likely take one year or longer to see a specialist. I would be put onto a waiting list and they'd call when they had an opening.

"One year?!" I gasped.

I couldn't believe what I was hearing. This was urgent! I was in acute pain. My window to have a child felt like it was closing quickly. I was scared. I was desperate. I was powerless. My ability to manage my pain and the possibility of ever conceiving a child were wholly held in Dr. Mustache's unconcerned hands.

Dr. Mustache explained that my case wasn't considered to be urgent because the tumors were likely benign, I wasn't going to die from the condition, and my pain could be managed with a simple painkiller.

"You're not listening to me!" I cried in exasperation. "I take Advil. I've tried everything I can think of to ease my pain. It's incessant. I can't go on like this. I can't stand the pain anymore.

Please! Please help me! You've got to do something! I can't wait a year!" I sobbed desperately. Tears flowed freely down my cheeks.

Dr. Mustache, startled by my outburst, passed me a tissue. "You could try pairing one Advil with one Tylenol," he suggested. "Period pain and cramping is part of being a woman," he professed, "You're just upset right now. Go home and relax."

I was dumbfounded.

I couldn't think clearly to ask any more questions. I nodded and agreed, barely listening to the doctor's continuing platitudes. His dismissal of my pain and my concern was inexcusable. He implied that my discomfort was in my head and portrayed me as a hysterical woman, desperate for a baby—irrational to obvious solutions such as taking a painkiller. He did not ask any follow up questions about my symptoms nor did he refer me on to a gynecologist who might have been more knowledgeable about women's health and could have seen me within a reasonable timeframe. His shoddy medical practice left me powerless and losing hope that I could ever find relief from my pain or eventually conceive.

I escaped to my car and wept.

As my tears subsided, fear and anger set in. I believed that my case was absolutely urgent. It was my fertility, my promise to my husband, my fundamental purpose as a woman, my hopes, my dreams… my life. But to my doctor, and apparently to the medical system, my case wasn't urgent because it wasn't life threatening. It didn't matter that Advil, Tylenol, Midol, or any combination of painkiller was totally ineffective or that I could barely function through my day because of the searing pain. It wasn't cancer—or so Dr. Mustache assumed.

Walking out of the clinic that day, I knew in my heart that it was over. My hopes and dreams of becoming a mother would not be fulfilled. I could not have children. It was a shocking reality and one I would not fully believe or accept for years to come. But I knew. I decided not to share with Hoyt either my fears or the conviction with which I felt them creeping up and washing over me. I would be positive and hope and plan right along with my husband. It couldn't be the end for us. Our quest for children was surely not over.

Hoyt and I tried to be positive, to look on the bright side of things. I could wait and see a specialist, have surgery, and then we'd be back in the baby making business. It sounded simple enough. Well, it didn't turn out to be quite that simple. A year is a long time to wait to see a gynecologist. I had so many questions but nowhere to find answers, leaving my imagination and my Google searches to run wild. I self-diagnosed until I was sure I had cancer or some other equally awful disease.

The pain I had month after month was debilitating. I spent endless days in bed after sleepless nights of trying to endure my pain. Handfuls of painkillers, heating pads, and warm baths did nothing to combat my agony. Even through the pain, I convinced myself that waiting for the gynecologist was my only option.

Chapter 3

My husband is a rancher, a prairie boy, and a cowboy at heart. Hoyt grew up on his family farm, learning to work the land and to ranch. As a young man, he took over the role of running the farm—a right of passage, passed down from the patriarchs before him. Hoyt operated his ranch while simultaneously working in the oilfield. He would work his two-week shift on his drilling rig and then come home to tend to his ranching duties. For ten years— from the time he graduated high school until two years into our marriage—Hoyt juggled working away and ranching. It was difficult to manage both careers at once, but we were fortunate to have my father-in-law, Doug, close by to help when Hoyt was away. As time went on, Hoyt and I both agreed that being apart for two weeks at a time was too hard. We were planning to start our family soon and we were in a financial position that no longer required Hoyt to work both jobs. Hoyt made the decision to resign from his lucrative drilling position to ranch full-time.

Cattle ranching is Hoyt's passion. Whether I wanted it to be or not, soon his passion became mine. From the first time I visited at his ranch, cows were a significant part of our life.

Our first weekend together included checking on the cows in the pasture, riding in the tractor while Hoyt cut hay, and helping Hoyt to move his tractor from one field to the next. I soon came to realize that sharing farm life with me was Hoyt's truest expression of love. He wanted me to love the ranch as much as he did.

As a teenager and even into my young adulthood, I had vowed never to marry a farmer. I thought I was a city girl at heart. I loved trips to the city, shopping, and fashion. Growing up on a farm, I knew the sacrifices and the labour it took to work the land. I disliked yard work, gardening, bugs, and dirt. I dreamed of the day that I could grow up, move to the city, and leave farm life behind.

How quickly my opinion would change.

There was something about the sparkle in Hoyt's eye when he shared his vision for his ranch that drew me to him. I wanted to share in his vision. I appreciated his perseverance and the sacrifices he had made in his young life to keep his family farm in the Colven name. He was honouring his family legacy—a value that had been instilled in me, too. As Hoyt shared his love of ranching with me, I could see our future together. Talk of children and expanding the ranch filled our conversations. I was deeply in love with this prairie boy—no teenage proclamations would stop my heart from loving him.

Eventually, my role on the ranch extended from packing lunches that would be eaten on the tractor or washing dusty work clothes. One day, Hoyt invited me to come out to the corrals with him to watch as he worked. I was amazed at his skills. He could anticipate which direction the cow would go and he could identify the calf that belonged to each cow without checking their matching tag numbers. I happily watched from the rail fence while Hoyt worked in the warm spring sunshine. He found cow-calf pairs easily and directed them to the appropriate pen, where they would wait to be hauled out to pasture.

Toward the end of the afternoon, Hoyt asked me to watch a gate. Watching a gate means standing in the middle of a 16-foot hole in the fence and stopping the cows from going out the gate. I was terrified of those 1300-pound beasts! I wondered how I should get them to stop. Ask them nicely, perhaps? I stood anxiously at the gate, praying that the cows wouldn't come close to me and bracing myself in case they did. The cows must've been just as scared of me as I was of them. They kept their distance, much to my relief.

I had passed my first unofficial test as a ranch wife—I had kept the cows in the corral. Now that my first experience with cattle had been a success, I was proving to Hoyt that I was willing to learn new skills and to work alongside him. We made a good team. I was ready to learn more about the cattle industry and what it took to make a family farm run successfully.

Hoyt took great pride in teaching me about ranching. The premise of our business is simple. In the spring, we send the cows and their calves out to pasture. Once there, the cows raise their calves and are bred by our bulls. They enjoy the summer, grazing in the coulees of our prairie pastures. In the fall, we round the cattle up and haul them back to the ranch. We sell the calves at an auction market in mid-October. The mother cows continue to graze until the weather gets too cold. Then they rest comfortably in corrals and small paddocks near our yard until they give birth again in the early spring. This cycle repeats each year. If a cow turns up open—not pregnant—in the fall, she gets a one-way ticket on a trailer ride to town and to the feedlot. Infertility is not an option on a successful cattle ranch. I was starting to see a parallel between our cows and me. Infertility was simply not an option. I anxiously waited for my appointment with the gynecologist to come as this parallel ran through my mind.

Chapter 4

That spring, my sister Rhonda finished her post-secondary training. Our whole family went to see her graduate as a Registered Veterinary Technician and to celebrate her milestone. I went, too, but I was in so much pain I could barely stand up despite taking far more than the recommended number of painkillers.

Halfway through my sister's celebratory dinner, my mom demanded I go to the emergency room. She insisted it wasn't typical to be in that much pain. I refused; I still thought the pain was "normal." I had recently been to see Dr. Mustache and he claimed I was just fine and should wait to see the specialist. He told me to take an Advil if I was in pain, so no, I was not going to the emergency room. My mom, however, is a force to be reckoned with when it comes to someone she loves. She doesn't take no for an answer, especially when it comes to health.

My mom believes in second opinions and more than one option to solve a problem. She can also outlast me when it comes to being stubborn, so we went to the emergency room. Our first stop was a large hospital downtown. The hospital parking lot was full, so we found a spot on a nearby side street and parked. We walked the short distance—me clutching my left side and staggering a step behind my mom—and finally arrived to find a packed waiting room and an ambulance screaming up to the doors.

After determining that it would be a five hour wait to see a physician, I decided I was not staying. I reminded my mom that my pain was "normal." I stubbornly stated that I was going back to my sister's celebration and left the waiting room. At some point on our walk back to the car, Mom convinced me to try a different hospital. Sometimes admitting defeat is easier than arguing, so I went.

After a quick trip across the city to a second, smaller hospital, we easily found a parking spot in the emergency room lot, close to the door. We spent two hours in the expansive reception area— my mom calmly waiting, me clutching my abdomen in unrelenting pain. Finally, my name was called and it was my turn to see the emergency room physician. I went in with trepidation and I came out with prescription painkillers and a referral for a gynecologist— someone I could see in two short weeks. It turns out the emergency room doctor was just as horrified by a one-year wait to see a specialist for my painful condition as was I.

This referral would eventually lead me to my new doctor, the opposite of Dr. Mustache. Competent and knowledgeable, she would tell me the truth every step along the way—even when it was a hard truth to hear. I would grow to have complete trust in her. That unwelcome trip to the emergency room with my mom was aligned by the Universe to bring Dr. Straight Shooter into my life.

Relief flooded my whole body. Relief from my physical pain thanks to my new painkillers. Relief from my emotional pain thanks to my referral slip. I left the hospital that day with a renewed sense of hope that this new doctor would hear my concerns and find the cause of my pain and infertility. A weight of worry had been lifted from my shoulders. I felt certain that Dr. Straight Shooter would know how to proceed on my journey to motherhood.

I shared my relief with my mom as we drove through the busy city streets and when we arrived back at my sister's party, Mom and I sat in the car for a moment before we headed back in to celebrate. She surprised me with a charm for my bracelet. It was a silver ball with pink sparkle letters that spelled HOPE. I wore that charm on my bracelet every day to remind myself to choose to hope.

You will need an abundance of hope and resilience on this journey of infertility. Sometimes I wasn't strong enough to hope, but Hoyt was, or my sister was, or my family was. Choose hope, even when things seem hopeless. Lean on the people around you to hope when you can't seem to do it for yourself. Be brave.

Chapter 5

Two weeks later, I found myself sitting in Dr. Straight Shooter's office waiting and wondering what the appointment would bring. I was mesmerized by the models of fetuses at different stages inside the womb that adorned Dr. Straight Shooter's exam room. I was studying them so intently that the soft knock on the door startled me as my doctor entered.

The small, fashionably dressed woman introduced herself with a firm handshake. She asked me why I was there and about my medical history. I took a shaky breath and my story came tumbling out. I tried to convey how fearful I was that the tumors in my uterus were cancerous or that I would not be able to have a baby.

Dr. Straight Shooter listened intently, asking questions about my symptoms as I talked. When I had shared my symptoms and concerns, she reviewed the medical records that had been sent from Dr. Mustache's office.

"Let's take a look and see what's going on," she said.

I laid down on the bed and tried to relax as Dr. Straight Shooter lowered the lights and examined me with the aid of an ultrasound machine. "I see two tumors. The larger one is 8 cm in length. The second tumor is 5 cm in length. Uterine fibroids are quite common, but they can be painful and they can cause infertility."

The lights came on and I sat up with a lump in my throat and a sinking feeling in the pit of my stomach. "Will I be able to have a child?" I asked, my voice thick with emotion.

Dr. Straight Shooter sat down slowly and made eye contact. She took a deep breath, "I don't know the answer to that. I will know more when I can remove the tumors and see what damage has been done. Right now, my concern is to address the cause of your pain. I'm prescribing a medication designed to shrink uterine fibroids and painkillers to manage your pain. I'm also putting you onto a wait list for surgery. It will be a six-week wait for a surgery date. After surgery, we can make a fertility plan."

I felt numb and nodded robotically.

That wasn't the cheery and hopeful answer that I was hoping for, but it was honest. I left the office that day feeling like Dr. Straight Shooter had heard my concerns and was honest about my condition. She was knowledgeable and capable. I appreciated her immensely.

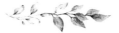

My surgery was scheduled for mid-February—right in the middle of calving season. Calving means checking cows every four hours, in all kinds of weather, and dealing with unexpected situations. Seconds count and can mean life or death for a baby calf. Calving is not a time you can be away for a few days without serious repercussions. This calving period would be one of the many times we would turn to our family for support and a helping hand. My sister-in-law, Dixie, who can do anything including driving a tractor, assisting a calving, and handling cows quietly and competently, agreed to come to take care of our cattle so Hoyt could be with me when I went for surgery.

The day of the surgery finally came and I was ready. I had imagined I would be walking into something akin to the set of *Grey's Anatomy* where Meredith would be my doctor and have something reassuring to say in a monologue before surgery. It turns out, Meredith wasn't there, much to my disappointment. It was bright and cold in the operating room and the only speech I heard was the anaesthesiologist counting backward from ten.

My last and only surgery had occurred when I was six and my tonsils were removed. I remember waking up wanting Jell-O. This time I woke up and wanted Hoyt, but he was not there. I couldn't feel my legs. I thought I was paralyzed. The pain from my surgery was overwhelming. Fortunately, the feeling of paralysis was just due to compression stockings put on to prevent blood clots, and when they were taken off, the feeling came back to my legs. A morphine drip helped dull the pain from my surgery.

The pain in my heart, however, was just about to begin.

Dr. Straight Shooter came in shortly after I woke up to tell me how the surgery went. The surgery had taken seven hours in total to complete—three hours longer than expected. I fought through the fogginess of the anesthesia to listen and understand as my doctor explained.

"I was able to remove the tumors successfully, but, unfortunately, there is an unexpected complication."

I braced myself as Dr. Straight Shooter continued.

"During the surgery, I discovered Stage 4 endometriosis which means that scar tissue and endometrial tissue have grown and covered many of your internal organs—including your ovaries, oviducts, bladder, and intestines."

I laid in shocked silence.

I had heard the word *endometriosis* once before, years earlier while overhearing my mom on the phone with a friend. I had no idea what that word meant. I just knew it must be bad.

Dr. Straight Shooter continued, "The good news is, I was able to remove most of the endometrial tissue. The bad news is, it will grow back in time. There is considerable scarring and damage to your ovaries and uterus. A piece of surgical mesh is holding your uterus together where the larger tumor once was. It will grow into the wall of your uterus as you heal. You will need the help of a fertility doctor to conceive because the scarring and damage from the endometriosis is so extensive. Call my office and schedule a follow up appointment in six weeks. We can talk more then."

When my doctor left, I was alone in my hospital room with nothing but hot tears running down my face and the slow movement of the hands on the clock to mark the passing of the day as I tried to imagine what this news meant for me.

I would never be able to conceive without assistance.

Those words were not welcome in my hospital room or my head, let alone in my heart. As the reality of Dr. Straight Shooter's diagnosis started to sink in, the pink sparkles on my hope charm were a little less sparkly with every breath I took.

Chapter 6

Once I had returned home from the hospital and started to heal—body and heart—the word *endometriosis* became familiar on my tongue as I said it so often. I researched and investigated the disease. According to Health Canada's website, endometriosis is a common condition affecting one in six women. It's a condition in which endometrial cells, similar to the cells found inside the uterus, grow outside of the uterus—often around the oviducts, ovaries, bowel, or bladder. Endometrial tissue acts similarly to the tissue found inside the uterus. Estrogen causes this tissue to grow, thicken, and attempt to shed with each menstrual cycle. Since the tissue has no way of leaving the body, it causes adhesions, scarring, implants, and lesions. The lesions become inflamed and swollen, often leading to debilitating pain and in some cases, infertility.

Pain and infertility are two of the primary symptoms of endometriosis—at least in my case they were. I experienced all manner of pain—pelvic pain, cramping, back pain, sciatic pain, pain during sex, pain during bowel movements. Other symptoms I endured included heavy, long-lasting and intensely painful periods, clotting, and of course—difficulty conceiving a child.

Interestingly, the stage of endometriosis does not necessarily correspond to the severity of pain a woman may experience. For example, if there are endometrial lesions near your sciatic nerve, as there were near mine, you may experience pain radiating down your thigh. The severity of pain is directly related to the placement of the lesions and scarring.

Endometriosis is difficult for doctors to diagnose. I first remember experiencing unbearable pain with my period as a thirteen-year-old girl. I was diagnosed with endometriosis at age twenty-six. Receiving a diagnosis of endometriosis can be a long and frustrating process. This condition is poorly understood and there are no known ways to prevent its development.

If you are experiencing symptoms that are synonymous with endometriosis, talk with your doctor and advocate for further investigation into what might be causing your symptoms. Hopefully it won't take thirteen painful years for you to finally receive your diagnosis as it did for me.

Chapter 7

Growing up, summers were busy. We worked hard, labouring together as a family to do what needed to be done on the farm. My brother and I had many responsibilities, even at a young age. While my friends were swimming or away at summer camp, I was pulling weeds and doing laundry.

My dad would often reward us for a day of hard work with a short drive in our little blue van to our small town, for ice cream at a shop aptly named *Sweet Temptations*. We would ride in the back seat, fighting as only siblings do. The ice cream shop seemed to have a million flavors—bubble gum, maple walnut, black cherry. You name it; they had it all. It was a sweet reward at the end of a hot and busy day.

Every summer, the fair came to the capital city of our province. I would see the commercials on TV and hear my friends share their excitement about the fair. If we drove by the fairgrounds—likely on our way to somewhere much less interesting—I could see the rides and hear the music. The intrigue of the carnival games, the smell of mini-donuts, the excitement of the flashing, colourful lights, and the beat of the music from the main stage were almost too much for a farm kid like me.

We never went to the fair as a family. It was expensive, and for my workaholic parents, the idea of crowds, cranky kids, and blazing sun was utterly unappealing when weighed against knowing they could be at home getting much needed work done. In the days following, I would listen to my friends talk about the fun they had had at the fair. I could not help but feel as if I was missing out on something.

So, it wasn't until I was twenty-six that I rode my first rollercoaster. I was apprehensive. I am a play-it-safe kind of girl, and amusement rides are what I would consider veering into danger. However, my brother, sister, and sister-in-law were all going, so I gave in to peer pressure and climbed aboard the *Galaxy Orbiter* at the West Edmonton Mall.

I told myself it couldn't be too dangerous or scary since children rode on it. I told myself that I could manage one trip around the track. I was strapped in and holding on extra tight. The ride started slowly and with a gentle rise. I thought to myself, *This is nice.* As we inched closer to the top of the first crest, I started to get a bit panicky. It was really high. The car stopped for a moment, teetering. I waited, wondering what would happen next. Was this the excitement that I had been missing out on each summer at the fair?

Then it happened.

The rollercoaster plummeted down the track, pushing me back in my seat and making my head hurt. I wanted off that rollercoaster—and fast—but I was strapped in, and the ride was far from over. I was terrified that I wouldn't be able to hold on tight enough and that I would fall out of the car. I hated the feeling of being pushed back with the gravitational force of the ride as air rushed past my face. I felt more and more nauseated. We careened up and down, twisting and turning, and seemingly out of control. When I thought I could not take another turn, there was a twist, an unexpected spiral, another sudden drop. My heart was pounding, my head was aching, and my breath was frozen in my chest. I jumped off the ride when it finally rolled to a stop at the gate, woozy and wobbly. I was resolved never to set foot on a wild and reckless rollercoaster ride again.

Infertility is like that—a rollercoaster of emotions. Each month starts the same way, filled with excitement and anticipation of a positive pregnancy test and ultimately—a child. When the long-awaited positive does not come, that once euphoric sense of anticipation is replaced with devastation and sorrow. The cycle of anticipation and excitement followed by devastation and sorrow is repeated again and again.

Infertility is messy and confusing and out of control. There's no guide book for infertility. A Google search didn't provide any of the answers I so desperately wanted either. Infertility permeated my life. Finances, marriage, friendships, social life, family, self-esteem, purpose, physical health, mental health, sex life—they were all affected by my infertility.

Yet, I suffered this unspoken sorrow quietly, privately.

Month after month, I continued to track, to schedule, to wait. I endured the dreaded "Two Week Wait" to discover if I was finally pregnant. I found myself standing in my bathroom with a pregnancy test in hand, more times than I can count. I would stare at my weary face in the mirror as I waved the stick slowly over the sink. Only one line would ever appear. I would squint and shake the pregnancy test harder, willing the other line to appear.

It didn't.

These moments stand still, the pinnacle of hope on my rollercoaster before my car plummets down to the lowest low. One moment followed by twists and turns that make my heart pound, my stomach churn, and my head spin.

So much for my no more rollercoaster rule; I was on a ride that I desperately wanted to escape, but I had to hold on extra tight because it seemed that there was simply no other option.

Chapter 8

Our decision to meet with the fertility doctor and proceed with IVF was an easy one for us. We had no other choice if we wanted to be parents. One year had passed since my surgery to remove my uterine fibroids and endometriosis. I had healed both physically and emotionally. Resilience and courage welled up inside of me. Hoyt and I had sacrificed to save enough money for the expensive and necessary fertility treatments. We had a window to try for that sweet baby we so badly wanted and I was ready to try again.

Shortly after Hoyt and I were married, my mom gave us two apple trees which we proudly planted in front of our house. In between the trees was a beautiful flower box my father-in-law had made for me with reclaimed wood from our barn. The barn is original to the property, built in the early 1900s. The land had been in the Colven family for years. Hoyt had recently completed minor renovations to the barn, leaving a pile of charmingly weathered barn wood boards just waiting to be repurposed into beautiful new items.

I commissioned my father-in-law to design and build the rustic flower box with the wood. It was the perfect shabby-chic addition to our front yard. I positioned the box between our apple trees and planted tulip bulbs underneath the trees. Finally, I circled the trunks of the trees with stones from the field behind our house. Those trees, the flower box, the rocks—to me they signified family, tradition, hope, and the future.

My grandma had large apple trees in her garden with lily-of-the-valley planted underneath. Each summer, Grandma and I would pick pail after pail of apples while the intoxicating floral scent floated through the air. We took the apples home to Grandma's kitchen to make applesauce, canned apples, and apple pie. I loved the delicate pink blossoms in the spring, the crisp, juicy fruit in the summer, and the mouth-watering scent of apple pie wafting from the oven in the fall. These memories were reminders of a happy childhood, the safety of my grandma's kitchen, and a simpler time in my life. I longed to pick apples with my children, creating memories to tuck away for later.

For three years, our trees did not produce apples and I had almost given up hope that they would ever bear fruit. The week before our first round of fertility treatments was to begin, I was walking down the lane with our dogs when something caught my eye. There, on our previously barren tree, was a small, pink apple.

I stared at that apple with disbelief.

The tree was no longer barren; finally, it was bearing fruit. I was overjoyed and took this little apple as a sign from Heaven. Surely this was a sign that I, too, would soon bear fruit. It was the sign I needed to reassure me that everything would work out. It was my sign that I had made the right decision to pursue fertility treatments. It was my sign that the needles, the travelling, the expense, the appointments—they would all be worth the effort. It was my sign that soon, I would be a mother. I hurried back to the house to tell Hoyt that the Universe was on our side. My heart was buoyed with hope, ready to face whatever challenges fertility treatments would throw my way.

Chapter 9

Hoyt and I approached our fertility treatments with precision. We had planned. We had prepared every detail within our control. We had done our research and we had a strategy. Thousands of dollars in fees were paid, the dates were set. We were in. We were focused. All our energy—and money—was ready and waiting for this most important appointment. We were at the top of the rollercoaster, feeling full of promise and hope.

We made our way up to the fourth floor of the modern office building where the fertility clinic was located. We checked in, and waited. The room was full of other bright-eyed, wistful-looking mothers-to-be and anxious, slightly bored-looking husbands who were scrolling through farm equipment sites on their phones (okay, maybe that was just my husband, but you get the picture). We took our seats amongst the other restless couples to wait. Finally, our names were called and it was our turn to go and meet our fertility doctor.

These appointments always start the same: an internal ultrasound. There were small change rooms just outside the exam room. I slipped into an available room and quickly removed my pants and underwear. I wrapped the provided paper sheet around my bottom half. As I was changing, I couldn't help but notice the inspirational clichés such as *Live, Love, Laugh* and *Dance Like No One is Watching* printed in cheery colors on the shower curtain that was meant to offer privacy.

It struck me just how incongruous these contrived sayings were when juxtaposed against the seemingly insurmountable obstacle of infertility. I rolled my eyes at the attempt at privacy with the flimsy shower curtain when in a few short minutes I would be laying under a paper sheet with my feet in stirrups as Dr. Lucky Strike, an ultrasound tech, and the head nurse Evelyn examined, measured, charted, and tested the limits of my uncooperative reproductive system.

Hoyt was already seated on a chair in the corner of the small exam room. I smiled weakly at him as I entered. He reached out and gave my hand a reassuring squeeze as I hesitantly sat down on the ultrasound bed. I told myself, "Just lie back and relax," as if that would somehow slow my rapidly beating heart.

The room was dimly lit in order for Dr. Lucky Strike to see the ultrasound screen more clearly. I slowly relaxed and let the darkness of the room and the whirs and hums of the machines cocoon around me, lulling me into a semi-state of calm. My trust was now entirely in the hands of the fertility gods. My team of medical professionals was cheerful, but I had been through enough doctors' appointments by this point to know when something was amiss.

An unnerving silence settled over the room.

Dr. Lucky Strike whispered something to the tech who diligently wrote it in my file. That moment is frozen in time. It was that moment just before I plummeted into the dark. I felt that old familiar feeling of panic and dread. I could feel a lump forming in the back of my throat—the one I try to swallow but ultimately know will lead to tears. Much to my dismay, the tears came, even before I knew what was wrong.

The lights came on, and the exam was over, just like that. The paper sheet rustled as I fumbled to sit up on the exam bed. I looked at Hoyt and he stared back at me, speechless. Fear and uncertainty sat in the room like the proverbial elephant. Dr. Lucky Strike directed me to dress and meet in his office when I was ready. Evelyn finished the notations she was writing and carried my chart full of bad news away to file as the ultrasound tech sent me a pitying look and fled out of the exam room behind Dr. Lucky Strike. Hoyt and I were alone for a moment in the empty exam room.

The expression on my face must have betrayed my fear. Hoyt tried to reassure me. "It's going to be okay, honey. Whatever it is, we will figure it out. We always do. Get dressed and I'll see you in a few minutes." With that, Hoyt turned and walked down the hall to find Dr. Lucky Strike's office.

I shimmied to the privacy of the change room wrapped in my rustling paper sheet as gracefully as possible. I quickly dressed and tried to dry my tears. I took a deep breath to clear my head while reciting the inspirational quotes on the shower curtain to distract my racing thoughts. I walked slowly down the hallway, bracing myself for whatever news lay on the other side of my doctor's door. All the while thinking of that little pink apple on my tree—my sign of fertility.

I entered the office and took a seat next to Hoyt. My doctor smiled and began to debrief us on the exam.

"From what I see on the ultrasound, Janice, it appears as though your oviducts are blocked," Dr. Lucky Strike explained.

Oviducts are more commonly known as fallopian tubes. Oviducts were "discovered" by Gabriel Fallopian and were therefore named in his honor. In her book, *Heavy Flow*, Amanda Laird states that "the road to modern gynecology was paved with misogyny, racism, and abuse." She encourages that meaningful and useful descriptors should be used to describe a woman's anatomy. For this reason, I have chosen to use the descriptive term, oviduct.

"These blockages could possibly be a result of scar tissue or endometrial lesions that have attached to your oviducts. If the tubes are blocked, the fluid that would normally flow freely through them becomes trapped inside. It leaks back into the uterus because it has nowhere else to go. This becomes significant because it will wash any fertilized eggs out of your uterus leaving them far from the correct location for implantation. We need to investigate further using an HSG test before we can schedule fertility treatments of any kind."

I was stunned.

I heard Hoyt shift uncomfortably in his chair, muscles tight, gaze unwavering as he listened intently to the doctor explain the Hysterosalpingography (HSG) test. I tried—unsuccessfully—to fight down the ball of fear growing in the pit of my stomach. I clenched my fists in my lap as my nails bit into my skin and tried to stay in control of my emotions.

"An HSG test uses dye and an X-ray machine to look inside the oviducts. It will be performed at the hospital. I will give you medication to help you to relax. Then, I will inject dye into your uterus. From there, we can follow the dye with the X-ray to determine if your oviducts are allowing fluid to pass through freely or if they are blocked," Dr. Lucky Strike explained.

"What will be the next step if my oviducts are blocked?" I asked shakily.

"You'll require surgery to remove them if the HSG test shows that they are in fact blocked," my doctor replied. "I will book the HSG test to be done next week."

I hung my head, feeling defeated. I had just spent a whole year recovering from surgery and the thought of enduring another major procedure was upsetting. IVF was not even an option until we knew if my oviducts were functioning. We shook Dr. Lucky Strike's hand and turned to leave the room.

It was a difficult walk back through the waiting room. I am sure every woman there was thanking her lucky stars that she was not the one leaving in tears. It would be only the first of many tearful walks through this waiting room for me.

As we left the clinic, the receptionist gave me a look as if I was a child whose dog had just run away. Pity. The look—as if I did not feel bad enough—was accompanied by a cheerful and unwelcomed, "Okaaayyy, thanks for coming in! See you soon!"

I felt blindsided by the fact that my body had seemingly failed me again. I was frustrated that my oviducts were hijacking my fertility. I had just recovered from the myomectomy to remove my uterine fibroids and excision to remove my endometrial lesions. The idea of more tests and another surgery made my vision narrow while the room began to spin. "Deep breaths, hang on," I urged myself.

Bit by bit, I was losing more and more of my fertility and my womanhood. I was distraught. I felt powerless to change or control anything that was happening with my fertility.

I was struck by the complexity of my body. There was so much more to conceiving a child than the basics revealed in a simple Google search. That complexity scared me. How could I possibly control all the intricate inner workings of my reproductive system? Would it be possible for my doctor to regulate and control each facet enough for me to actually conceive? How much longer would it be before my dreams of conception became a reality?

Hoyt walked me to the truck, held my hand while I cried, sympathized with my "It's not fair!" rant, and took me home to pick up the pieces. So much for my belief in signs from Heaven.

Chapter 10

My HSG test showed that my oviducts were in fact blocked, just as Dr. Lucky Strike had predicted.

"Surgery is our best option at this point," he told me one week later at our follow up appointment. "Your oviducts are not serving you any longer. They aren't functioning as they should. In fact, they're likely contributing to your ongoing infertility," he reasoned.

I was referred back to Dr. Straight Shooter, who agreed with the diagnosis of blocked oviducts and the recommendation for surgery to remove the offending pieces of my womanhood.

"Let's get you in as soon as possible," Dr. Straight Shooter said, as I signed the surgery consent forms. I agreed completely. The sooner I could have the surgery, the sooner my plan would be back on track.

I could do one more surgery if it meant taking one step closer to my baby, I reasoned. In those rare, quiet moments that I found myself alone with my thoughts, tears would often stream down my cheeks, unchecked. At night when I tried to fall asleep, when I was driving home after work, or when I was in the shower, my tears would fall. They had to escape. It took every ounce of will power and energy to keep my tears at bay and my emotions regulated during the day. My heart couldn't hold my tears or my sorrow for one second longer when I was alone.

Eventually, my tears subsided as days turned into weeks. Time had a way of making my heart hurt less. I could breathe again. *Why me?* turned into *Okay, I can do this. I will do this!*

My surgery, a bilateral salpingectomy, was scheduled for March 17th, St. Patrick's Day. It had been eight weeks since Dr. Lucky Strike, my fertility doctor, had delivered the news that my oviducts needed to be removed. Eight weeks since I had been referred back to Dr. Straight Shooter, my gynecologist. Soon, Dr. Straight Shooter would remove both of my offending oviducts. With any luck, this surgery would increase my chances of sustaining a pregnancy.

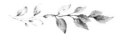

Parent-Teacher Conferences for my grade two families were scheduled the evening before I was to have surgery. I spent the day prior to the conferences in a frenzied cloud of activity as I tidied the classroom, helped my students clean their desks, and made sure that each child's learning portfolio was complete and in order. I mentally ticked items off of my to-do list as the hands on the clock swept around the face dramatically faster than usual—or so it seemed.

At 4:00 pm, parents and children started arriving for their appointed time slots. The school was buzzing with a whirlwind of excited children and families coming and going to meet with teachers throughout the school.

I welcomed families, shared progress and concerns, and had crucial conversations throughout the evening. I was glad to have reading scores and classroom behavior to focus on the night before my surgery. It kept my busy brain from worrying. That particular year, I had a challenging class with extreme behaviors that had left my fragile heart empty and my energy sapped. I was ready to hand over my class to a substitute teacher for six weeks while I had my oviducts removed and I recovered at home. I was ready to focus on getting healthy and preparing my body for my baby.

Hoyt and I arrived at the hospital bright and early on March 17th. As I waited in line at the admitting desk, I ruminated over how disappointed I was to be missing St. Patrick's Day with my students. I had purchased a sparkly green hat and shamrock inspired accessories to wear. I had planned to serve shamrock sugar cookies at story time while I read leprechaun tales aloud to the class.

"Instead," I grumbled to myself, "I am here, about to have surgery."

I signed the consent documents and double checked my personal information. The admitting nurse put the hospital band around my wrist, making my impending surgery suddenly feel very real. I was back at the hospital once again. This time I knew what to expect and surgery did not seem as scary as the first time around.

Hoyt waited with me in my pre-op room. He kept the mood light with his witty banter and impish smile. A nurse appeared in the doorway to walk me to the operating room. Hoyt came as far as he could, then hugged me and watched me walk down the hallway.

Once again, I found myself in a bright, cold operating room, staring into the eyes of the anesthesiologist as he counted back from ten and I drifted into a deep sleep.

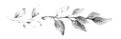

The face of my recovery room nurse slowly came into focus as I tried to fight my way to the surface of consciousness.

"Janice, you're in recovery, wake up, your surgery is finished and everything went well," she explained as she tried to rouse me.

Images became sharper as I fought the temptation to slip back into sleep. I could feel the compression stockings forcing a rhythm on my unappreciative legs. I caught a whiff of antiseptic wash as I took a shallow breath. I could feel the muted bite of pain in my abdomen. I made out the constant drip, drip, drip of my IV pump from somewhere beside my bed. I squeezed my eyes shut against the bright, florescent lights above me as my nurse continued to check my vital signs and bustle around the recovery room.

Everything went well—it's over, I whispered to myself as the drugs pulled me under and I drifted back to a dark and dreamless sleep.

"I successfully removed both oviducts. They had been badly damaged by scar tissue," Dr. Straight Shooter reported early the next morning. "Go home and recover. Make an appointment with my office for a follow up in six weeks," she instructed as she signed my discharge papers.

"When can I start fertility treatments again?" I asked, anxious for her response.

"We can discuss that at your follow up appointment," my doctor cautiously responded. "I'll refer you back to the fertility clinic if you are healed and you can discuss a course of treatment then."

Relieved, I thanked Dr. Straight Shooter and settled back into my hospital bed. In six weeks, I would be healed. With renewed hope, I felt resilient and ready to tighten the straps and hold on. My rollercoaster car was gaining momentum once again. It was slowly crawling its way up the track to the precipice that I hoped and assumed would be my highest high.

I spent the night in the hospital and was discharged early the next morning. After leaving the hospital, I insisted to Hoyt that we stop for brunch. He cautioned that we still had a long drive ahead and that my pain medication would soon wear off which would make for an uncomfortable ride. Still sailing on whatever wonder drug I had been prescribed at the hospital, I promised that I would be fine. I yearned to feel "normal" and not as though I had just undergone another surgical procedure. I was determined that brunch was the perfect antidote. Hoyt finally relented and we ordered breakfast at a local restaurant.

The food tasted so flavorful and delicious after the bland and unappealing meals that had been delivered to my bedside table from the hospital kitchen. Pancakes topped with whipped cream on my plate and the scent of strong, hot coffee wafting from my mug was exactly what I craved. The hum of conversation, clanging of silverware against plates, and muted music in the background paired with the effects of my pain medications soothed me into contentment.

My spirits were buoyed by my doctor's assessment that I would heal in six weeks' time. I assumed that it would be a straightforward path from recovery to fertility treatments to pregnancy. My day-dreamy logic told me that we would need a bigger house once we were able to start our family. My Type A personality told me that we needed to start looking and planning—immediately. It seemed like a reasonably good idea to look at ready-to-move houses before leaving the city for the two-hour drive home. The idea was that we needed to (quickly before the painkillers wore off) pick out a bigger house that could be moved to our ranch, one with room for our future babies. Oviducts gone? Check! We were another step closer to our dream coming true.

Chapter 11

Six weeks later, I had healed from my surgery, and we were ready to try again, hopeful once more. Dr. Lucky Strike had given us the go-ahead to schedule a cycle of in vitro fertilization (IVF).

IVF is a method of assisted reproduction. Not long ago, IVF was a mysterious word and a little-known procedure that few infertile couples pursued. Today, IVF is common in Canada. In 2017, 33,000 cycles were initiated across our country. This is not surprising, as infertility affects one in six women. The number of IVF cycles and resulting live births continues to grow each year as Canadians learn more about the options available to infertile couples.

Some provinces such as Ontario and Quebec offer funding for fertility treatments. This opens opportunity for couples who would not otherwise be able to afford expensive fertility treatments. Saskatchewan, my home province, does not fund fertility treatments, but Hoyt and I were committed to seeing our dream through to fruition. We were willing and ready to use our life savings, credit cards, and loans to pay for our fertility treatments if it meant we could be parents.

The first step in my IVF cycle was to begin taking a traditional birth control pill. This seemed counterintuitive to my logical brain.

Dr. Lucky Strike had explained at our initial appointment before our IVF cycle was set to begin, "The hormones in the birth control will supress your natural hormones and your menstrual cycle. That will allow the fertility drugs to manipulate your ovaries to produce eggs and to thicken the lining of your uterus to accept an embryo." Whether it made sense to me or not, I did as Dr. Lucky Strike directed and dutifully swallowed my birth control pill every morning like clockwork for the month after our consultation appointment.

Hoyt and I arrived at the fertility clinic, eager to begin our long-awaited IVF cycle. I was ushered to the back for blood work and then to the ultrasound room while Hoyt waited in the reception area.

This time, I made it through the first ultrasound with no bad news, no lumps in my throat, and no tears in the waiting room. It was a small victory for an emotional girl like me. Maybe my reproductive system was finally ready to cooperate. Perhaps, finally, we had shown it who was boss. I went home with a pink bag full of fertility drugs, needles, alcohol swabs—and a Visa card that had been charged to the max.

We headed down the highway with a bag full of expensive drugs and supplies, ready to buckle ourselves into our baby rollercoaster ride once again.

Two hours later, I found myself standing in the bathroom with a needle hovering over my tender skin, paralyzed by fear. I can still feel the warm spring breeze on my skin, fresh from the open bathroom window. I can hear the hum of the bathroom lights. I can smell the freshly laundered towels that were hanging on the rack.

What was I thinking?!

My stomach flips and my vision gets fuzzy around the edges when I have my blood taken by a professional—when all I have to do there is stare at a dot on the ceiling and wait for it to be over.

It is all I can do to stay in the chair. How did I agree to stab myself with two very long, sharp needles twice a day?

After a long day in the city where his job was to keep his emotional wife in a state of semi-calm, Hoyt had fled to the sanctuary of the hay fields near our house. I am sure he was glad for the escape to his tractor for a few hormone-free hours of cutting hay.

I was on my own.

Going through fertility treatments revealed a strength I did not know I possessed. Needles are not for the faint-of-heart, but I was willing to do anything at this point to become a mother—so, scared or not, I closed my eyes and stabbed.

Prescription drugs, painful injections, trips to the city for ultrasounds and more medications, missed days at work, sleepless nights, expensive bills, and tear-soaked pillows—all badges of honor on my quest for a baby. I took it all with a fierceness that surprised me.

I was sure the stars were aligned in our favor this time. It had to work. I pleaded, bargained, promised, cried, and prayed. *Please, Lord, let it work this time.*

At first, the ultrasound appointments were spread out. As the cycle progressed, I went more and more frequently, until soon, I was wearing a path up and down the highway to that glamorous, expensive fertility clinic. By now, I was on a first-name basis with the nurses and technicians, chatting with them about their daily lives; it is almost inevitable as these women saw me in compromising situations such as wrapped in a paper sheet with my feet in stirrups. After each ultrasound, Dr. Lucky Strike would tell me how much my follicles had grown.

Follicles are small, fluid filled sacs found inside the ovaries. Each sac has the potential to hold and release an egg for fertilization. A successful round of IVF should result in a minimum of three mature follicles. Each follicle must be between sixteen and twenty millimeters in average diameter prior to ovulation in order to be viable.

7 mm, 5 mm, 8 mm, 6 mm. I had four follicles. That was enough. They were small but had the potential to grow. 8 mm, 8 mm, 10 mm, 9 mm. Progress—the drugs were working. That was good. 11 mm, 9 mm, 12 mm, 13 mm. Getting closer, almost there. 16 mm, 17 mm, 19 mm, 20 mm. Relief. The follicles grew, and they were full of eggs. I closed my eyes and breathed a sigh of relief, so grateful for what I thought was my body's positive response to the fertility drugs.

The appointments were surreal. Dr. Lucky Strike would tell me just enough to keep me hopeful, to keep the monsters in my head at bay. I was desperate for reassurance that my body was responding to the fertility drugs. More information, however, did not ease my anxiety. I simply could not relax or have confidence in the IVF process because of my past failed experiences with my reproductive system.

New worries and concern came with each new stage of my IVF cycle. At first, I worried whether my body would respond to the fertility drugs. Then I worried whether my follicles would grow to the appropriate size or if I would have enough follicles to make the cycle viable. Next I worried whether any of my eggs would mature sufficiently. My list of concerns and fears was endless. Knowing more or knowing less—neither scenario gave me peace.

Naively, blindly, I drove the long stretch of highway from our ranch to the city each morning, arriving at the clinic by 8:00 am sharp, for my daily blood work and internal ultrasound. Each day, I spent more money, missed more work, stabbed myself with another needle, and fell deeper in love with the dream of having a baby. I lived my days in a blur—half day-dream of what it would be like to finally feel our baby inside of me—half nightmare of what it would mean if this cycle of IVF failed and my womb remained empty.

Chapter 12

The end of June arrived and with it—a sense of relief. The school year was over. I could send this year's students on to the next teacher and look forward to a new group coming in the fall. When the school year had ended, my sister-in-law, Dixie, packed up her children and made the four-hour trip to our house. While Hoyt and I were in the city for fertility appointments, Dixie would help with haying. She would visit our pastures to check on our cows, making sure that they were healthy and safe. Dixie's presence gave Hoyt a sense of security, knowing that his sister would look after the cattle and the ranch while we were away.

I was almost done the most difficult part of my treatments—the needles, the early morning trips to the city, and the daily blood tests and ultrasounds. It was nearly time for my retrieval. I was eager to finally move on to the next phase.

The last step before the egg retrieval is what is called a "trigger shot." This shot is the important one, the one you cannot miss, the one you cannot forget, the one you cannot delay. The trigger shot contains human chorionic gonadotropin (hCG), which initiates ovulation and the release of the eggs from their follicles. This allows the doctor to suck the eggs out of the safety of the follicles and into the big, bright, sterile world of the embryology lab.

This embryology lab was where my eggs would be fertilized with Hoyt's sperm and the miracle of life would begin for our child. My trigger shot was set for 11:00 pm. I double and triple checked the time on the protocol sheet I had received from the fertility clinic. I wrote it on the calendar. I wrote the time on sticky notes and stuck them around the house. I set alarms. I was not going to make a mistake.

At 10:59 pm, I was standing in the kitchen, mixing drugs and filling the syringe. Three cell phones were lined up to make sure the time was right, my husband was beside me, and we were ready to go. As soon as the cell phone glow showed 11:00 pm, I was ready—one quick jab, and it was over. The chain reaction had started. My eggs were getting ready to release and soon become embryos. The wonder and magic of the whole process amazed me. To think, my babies were eggs in my follicles right now and they were about to begin their journey. My miracle babies. I could not wait to meet them and fell asleep dreaming of my sweet children.

The next morning, as usual, Hoyt was cool, calm, and collected. I, on the other hand, was emotional—but with a new twist—Ativan. This was the sedation medication that Dr. Lucky Strike had prescribed to relax me during the retrieval procedure. According to my protocol, I was scheduled to take the Ativan two hours prior to my arrival at the clinic. That meant putting the tiny pill under my tongue shortly after we left home that morning.

I don't remember much of the trip to the city that day. Hoyt recalls that I was emotional—weepy and fearful of failure one moment, dreaming on cloud nine of babies and nurseries the next.

When we arrived at the fertility clinic, Hoyt had to help me out of the truck and hold my arm while gently guiding me into the building and toward the reception area of Dr. Lucky Strike's office. My legs felt like jelly and refused to move on their own. My body was warm and everything seemed to be fuzzy and glowing. My thoughts came slow and jumbled and I collapsed gratefully into one of the waiting room chairs, relieved to be sitting down.

"Janice?" I heard Evelyn, the head nurse at the clinic, call my name. Hoyt helped me to my feet and Evelyn took my arm. I leaned on her and we started a slow and wobbly walk down the long hallway to a procedure room. There was a square window at the end of the hall. My attention was solely focused on the blue sky and sunshine beyond that window. Everything else closed in, black and fuzzy except for that window. I was floating along, walking on air to that sunshiny place.

Evelyn helped me change into a hospital gown, settled me into a vinyl recliner, and wrapped me in a warm blanket. She made pleasant conversation as sunlight streamed through the over-sized windows. From the cozy cocoon of my blanket, I could see the beautiful landscape of the city.

I watched as people hurried along the street, going about their errands, while I was moments away from participating in the miracle of life beginning. I considered the irony of my monumental day compared to the seemingly mundane activity of the people in the street below while Evelyn tightened a tourniquet and searched my bruised arm for a vein that might accept her needle.

My veins are small and often hard to find. Daily blood work over the last two weeks had left my arm sore, bruised, and my veins unwilling to cooperate. With a few tries, Evelyn was able to find a vein and start my IV—a precaution in the event of a complication during the retrieval procedure. I relaxed into the recliner, warm, dreamy, and decidedly detached from reality, thanks to the Ativan. I had nothing to do but wait.

"It's time to go, Janice. The doctor is ready for you. It's time for your egg retrieval," Evelyn announced, breaking into the lovely daydream of motherhood that was playing out in my head. She helped me up and guided my languid body and my IV pole to the retrieval room, a short distance away.

It was a small, dark room humming with machines. There was a big screen on the wall across from the bed with the stirrups. I climbed up, positioned myself in the stirrups, and waited. Evelyn told me that in a few minutes, if I watched the screen, I would be able to see my eggs coming out as they were retrieved. It was incredible. At that moment, all the money, needles, and mood swings in the world were worth it.

Dr. Lucky Strike entered the room wearing a full gown, hairnet, and mask. He explained that an internal ultrasound would guide him as he inserted a large needle through my cervix to puncture each follicle and remove the eggs from inside their sac. I laid still—my body relaxed. My gaze was intent on the screen. I ignored the pressure of the ultrasound and the needle as they entered my body. I felt the sharp stab of pain as the needle pierced my follicles.

I waited. I held my breath. I anxiously searched the screen for signs of my eggs. I waited more. I watched as slowly, a swirl of blood churned maliciously around the clear white field of the screen.

The room became quiet.

The joyful, expectant mood in that little room turned cold. I kept my eyes glued to the screen, watching for my babies, but they did not come. They wouldn't be coming because there were none. I saw blood dance around the screen: blood, but no eggs.

The doctor looked up and said the words I can still hear. "I'm sorry, but there are no eggs."

I did not understand. I could not process his words or their meaning. My vision blurred, and then Hoyt was there beside me. I could hear a sound, kind of a cry, kind of a scream, kind of a howl. It took me a minute to realize the sound was coming from somewhere deep within me. It was the unique sound of a heart that had just been shattered into a million pieces. It was as though I was floating above the scene, watching my life blow apart.

Evelyn walked me to the recovery room and settled me into a recliner. I couldn't stop sobbing. My outburst was probably upsetting all the other egg-bearing women and dampening the joy and expectancy of their own egg retrieval days. That recovery room was the scene of my unravelling for the 45 miserable minutes that I spent recuperating after my procedure—although time seemed to have stopped the moment that crimson swirls of blood appeared on the retrieval monitor. Hoyt sat beside me, holding my hand, unsure of what to say or how to comfort me while simultaneously trying to process what had happened.

Soon after my time in recovery had concluded, Evelyn handed Hoyt my discharge papers while she murmured platitudes that did nothing to offer comfort. She guided Hoyt and me through a maze of hallways to a door that led to the main hallway and elevator. My abdomen ached, my vision was clouded by tears, and my muscles were experiencing the lingering effects of the Ativan. My physical symptoms were nothing in comparison to the immeasurable pain in my heart. I felt like the devastating reality of my egg retrieval was something the clinic would rather keep secret—like my outcome was bad for business so they shuffled me out the back to avoid upsetting their potential clients who sat expectantly in the waiting room.

Evelyn told us to go home and rest—the receptionist would call with a follow up appointment. My husband took my hand, pushed the elevator button, held me on the ride down, gently placed me into the truck, and took me home to pick up the shattered pieces of my heart.

Chapter 13

Life may have stopped in one breath for me, but for the rest of the world, it was humming right along. While we drove home, I made the painful calls to my mom and to Darlene to let them know that my body had not responded to the fertility medications the way it should have and my follicles were empty.

"It didn't work. I can't give you a grandchild. I'm so sorry," I mournfully sobbed into the phone, first to my mom and then Darlene.

"That's ok, honey. Don't cry. You can try again, right?" Mom soothed. "Is it sunny there today? It sure is cloudy here. It might rain," she continued, trying to change the subject to something less emotionally charged.

My mom had no idea how to anticipate what I needed or what would possibly bring me comfort in the midst of my deep sorrow. She couldn't know. Infertility had never been her reality and it was difficult for her to imagine the enormity of my pain.

I mumbled a reply about the weather and made a quick excuse to end the call. My heart was broken. I didn't know if I could ever put my life back together or if I would survive the grief in my soul. I felt like I didn't have enough strength left to even take my next breath. I was trying unsuccessfully to process what this failed retrieval truly meant and what would happen, or not happen, as a result. The reality that I would not be a mother hit me.

I was angry and hurt. I needed comfort, love, and connection in this moment. To talk about the weather seemed so trivial and unimportant in contrast to the gravity of my situation.

It wasn't as simple as just trying again. We were not able, in that moment—or for many months to come—to consider attempting another round of fertility treatments. Hoyt and I needed time to grieve, to heal, and to process our loss. Financially, additional treatments would mean countless sacrifices. We had just spent thousands of dollars for this cycle of IVF and were left with nothing but the massive Visa bill. I had missed work. I had made the long, daily trips to our fertility clinic for two weeks straight. I had given myself painful injections and suffered mood swings and weight gain—side effects of the fertility hormones. Emotionally, trying again would require a strength from deep within that, at the moment, I didn't feel I possessed. I had poured every ounce of emotional and mental energy into this cycle and I felt totally depleted.

I had carefully navigated the twists and turns of my rollercoaster ride. I had climbed to the full height of the track and had hovered precariously at the highpoint for a moment—trying wildly to take in the view and enjoy the feeling of being on top of the world. The coaster car stopped long enough for me to let my guard down before it cruelly rushed over the precipice and plunged down with all my hopes and dreams to the dark bottom below.

I needed my mom to help me work through what had happened. I needed empathy. In that moment I needed my mom to say, "Honey, this is awful. I'm here with you. You're not alone. I haven't ever had to live through what you've been through today, but I know it's bad and I know it hurts. Right now, let's just get through this moment together, breath through it. I love you and I'm here. Tell me what you need right now. Would you like to talk about how you're feeling? Do you want me to just stay on the line with you? Do you want to let me go now and I'll check back with you in a few hours?"

But that wasn't how our conversation went.

Infertility is an uncomfortable topic to discuss. It takes courage and strength to be a part of a woman's support system during infertility. It can be difficult and uncomfortable to navigate the layers of emotion that are inevitable. Knowing what the "right" thing to say or do in each situation is difficult because, often, the experiences are so unfamiliar.

The tumultuous emotions that I experienced while deep in fertility treatments evolved from day to day. I can tell you that after living through years of infertility and rebuilding my life after infertility, that there are simply no right answers. There's no guide book for moms, sisters, and friends to read in order to handle each situation gracefully.

Keep in mind that your mom or your sister might not know how to best support you. Mine didn't. They'll likely say the wrong thing or assume that they understand what you're feeling or thinking. Mine did. Your loved ones are doing their best to comfort you and to understand what you're going through—just like mine were. I learned to ask for what I needed. I had to be clear with the type of support or involvement that I craved. I tried to remember that the women supporting me were coming from a place of love.

What would I have liked to have said to my mom that day? I would have told her that empathy and connection were what I craved, that I didn't need quick answers or for her to fix anything. I just needed her to honor my emotions and to let me take the lead with the sort of support I needed in that moment.

The months that followed my failed IVF cycle were incredibly difficult. Each day and each new phase in my healing required something different. Some days, I needed to cry and feel sad and I wished for my mom or my sister to sit with me and be with me both physically and emotionally. Other days, I needed to be angry and to rant about my unfair situation and I needed someone to connect to the intense feelings of injustice that were raging in my heart. Every so often, I needed a distraction or some mindless chitchat to keep my brain from wandering to my infertility. Some days still, I needed to keep my thoughts and feelings to myself because they felt too private to share.

At times during the months after my failed IVF cycle, my emotions were so intense that I didn't think I could manage them alone. I wish the women who loved me would have understood that in order to be my authentic self, I needed a safe space to process the dark feelings swirling in my soul instead of pushing them down deep inside. I needed the women who supported me to connect with my experience and not expect or prefer that I paste on a smile and be "fine." I simply wasn't fine.

While Hoyt and I were in the midst of our long battle with infertility and trying to start our family, our siblings were busy building their own families. My brother, Derek, had three children—a boy and two girls—Hayden, Raegan, and Maeva. His wife, Ashley, was pregnant with another baby girl.

On Hoyt's side of the family, his sister, Dixie, had two children—a boy and a girl—Alex and Wyatt. Hoyt's brother and his wife, were expecting their first baby, also a girl. Both of my sisters-in-law were due only a few weeks apart and our families excitedly awaited the births of these baby girls.

These children brought life, joy, and laughter to our families. My mom and Darlene both took their roles as "Grandma" seriously. It weighed heavy on my heart that my empty follicles meant I wasn't able to give the gift any time soon of another grandchild to either of these women who meant so much to me.

After making my difficult phone calls to share my continued infertility with my mom and Darlene, I settled back into my truck seat. I gazed out the window, tears streaming down my cheeks, and watched as the prairie landscape whizzed by my window in a blur.

Chapter 14

Hoyt continued to drive the long stretch of highway, bringing us back to our childless life. When we arrived home, we were greeted by a salesman delivering a piece of equipment we had bought a few weeks prior. Hoyt pulled himself together and walked across the yard to meet the sales rep. He talked to the gentleman, checked over the machine, and dealt with the paperwork. I did what any logical girl who is spaced out on Ativan and fentanyl would do—I jumped on the lawn mower and decided to cut grass. I buzzed along our front lawn with the thoughts—*It's all your fault, your body is broken, faulty, you let Hoyt down, you'll never be a mother*—running on repeat through my mind while rivers of tears flowed from my red and swollen eyes.

Soon, the sales rep was on his way and Hoyt was alone. He slowly walked across our yard and stopped me on my lawn mower, breaking me from my trance. He insisted I come inside—maybe because I could no longer see through my tears or maybe because the lines in the lawn were starting to get a bit crooked.

Once inside, I couldn't quit moving. Sobs escaped my throat as I paced back and forth with my arms wrapped around my aching and empty womb. In the kitchen, I angrily piled the sink full of breakfast dishes into the dishwasher. In the living room, I irritably arranged and rearranged a stack of magazines on the coffee table. In the laundry room, I stuffed a load into the washer. Emotion squeezed my chest so hard I could barely breathe. If I stopped moving, I cried harder. My heart felt like it was being strangled. I couldn't breathe. There was blinding pain in my head. I just wanted it to stop.

Tequila seemed to be a reasonable answer.

I brought the bottle down from our liquor cabinet, cut up a lemon, grabbed the salt, and headed to my bed, my sweet husband in tow. Hoyt wasn't as confident that tequila was a good idea. He was probably trying to live up to the "responsible adult required for discharge" section of my post-surgical care papers.

"Honey, I know you're upset, but I don't think tequila is the answer here. Remember the Ativan? You're not supposed to have any alcohol!" Hoyt tried to reason.

I ignored his caution and continued to our bedroom—bottle in hand. I was determined to numb my pain and Hoyt's sensible argument did little to slow me down.

"I don't care. My heart hurts too much. I want the pain to go away," I declared angrily over my shoulder as I continued down the hall to my sanctuary.

Hoyt followed me to our bedroom and hesitantly sat on the edge of our bed. I twisted the cap off the bottle, poured liquor into two glasses, and handed one to Hoyt. Silently, I raised my glass. Reluctantly, Hoyt raised his glass to meet mine in a toast that neither of us wanted to make.

Salt, shot, lemon. Salt, shot, lemon.

My heart still hurt, so I kept pouring. Soon I had a belly full of tequila, salt in my bed, and lemon wedges on the bedside table. I hadn't expected the effect tequila shots would have in combination with sedatives and painkillers in my mixed-up, crisis-mode, hormone-laden body. I started to feel the effects fast: a warm rosy glow, unresponsive muscles, fuzzy edges to the world, and a familiar tingle moving up my body.

Suddenly, I was starving. The tequila combined with my overwhelming mixture of emotions had left me ravenous. I stumbled to the kitchen to check the fridge for munchies but found nothing enticing. The cupboard? I dug to the far back corner of the cabinet and there it was—a bag of nacho chips and cheese dip. Perfect.

I ran back to our bedroom and ripped open the bag. I twisted the lid off the jar and started to dip chips frantically and munch like crazy, one chip right after another. Chip crumbs joined the salt in my bed as cheese sauce dribbled down my chin and onto my shirt.

When I couldn't eat another bite, I paused for a moment with the half empty chip dip jar still in my hand—and was overcome by red-hot rage. I was furious. How could this happen?! My body betrayed me; my ovaries were defective, broken, and useless. My body had cheated me and Hoyt out of parenthood and the life of which we'd dreamed. I had let my husband down. I was a failure. It wasn't fair! I screamed and cried.

Then something unexpected happened.

The open glass jar of cheese dip went sailing across our bedroom, bright orange sauce flying everywhere. The empty jar smacked against the wall and fell to the floor. I looked at Hoyt and he looked back at me, shocked. We sat in astounded silence—too shaken to move or to speak—until the moment was shattered by the sound of heavy footsteps on our stairs and the squeak of our back door opening.

It was my father-in-law, Doug.

Doug had been out working in the hay field with Dixie while we were in the city for my retrieval. Doug had innocently come to the house for a drink of water, or maybe to ask my husband a question. We had shared only the most basic details of the reason for our daily trips to the city so Doug had no idea of what we had been through earlier in the day.

When I heard Doug's footsteps coming up the stairs to our house, I rushed out to meet him, almost-empty tequila bottle in hand. I am certain my unsuspecting father-in-law didn't know what to think when I appeared on the deck and insisted he have a drink with me—straight from the bottle. I didn't drink; I had had enough. I demanded he finish the bottle. By now we were out of lemons, so he drank the tequila straight up. This empty bottle triumph was met with not one, but two unexpected hugs from a cheese-dip-covered, puffy-eyed daughter-in-law. I am sure Doug had no idea what was wrong with me, but he had the good sense not to ask.

As afternoon turned to evening, my sister-in-law and my niece and nephew returned home from the hay field, ready for supper. What they found when they returned was far from a nice family dinner, prepared and hot on the table. Instead, the kids found a snack in the cupboard while their auntie wept into their mom's lap.

I laid in my bed with my head cradled on Dixie's lap, sobbing inconsolably. I felt such a sense of guilt and kept apologizing over and over.

"It's all my fault, I'm sorry, I'm so sorry," I cried. Dixie stroked my hair and tried to soothe me, even though her words could not staunch the steady flow of tears from my swollen, blood-shot eyes.

I felt so guilty. I felt I had let everyone down—Hoyt, my mom, Darlene, Dixie, myself. The more I cried, the more reasons I found to blame myself. Hoyt wouldn't be able to carry on his family name or family farm—because of me. We couldn't give our parents another grandchild—because of me. We had wasted our money on this cycle of IVF and incurred debt—because of me. My list went on and on. I truly believed that my infertility was my fault. I felt a crushing sense of responsibility and remorse—guilt so heavy I couldn't bear to lift my head or open my eyes.

It *was* all my fault. Not in the sense that I had purposely destroyed my fertility, but in the sense that it was me and my broken body that was crushing our dream and wasting our money. The weight of that guilt was unbearable and would have consequences for my emotional well-being and my marriage in the months to come.

It is one thing to know something rationally in your head. Your head is easy to convince. It's the story that is written on your heart that is harder, nearly impossible, to rewrite. The story written on my heart was *this is all your fault, you are broken, and you don't deserve happiness after taking it away from your husband.* It would take months—and the help of a mental health professional—for me to chip away at those words and to write something softer and closer to the truth.

The next morning, I woke up. For a brief half-asleep moment, I didn't remember. I rolled over and snuggled further into my blankets, luxuriating in the warmth of my bed, when suddenly, it all came rushing back. Tears welled up in my eyes, and I pulled the covers over my head, wishing for the solace of sleep to return. The sound of birds chirping and the bright light of a brilliant summer morning penetrated the darkness. I forced myself out of bed. I had to face the day.

My young niece and nephew were excited. It was their summer holiday. We live close to the lake and we had promised Alex and Wyatt a day playing at the beach. I was to be their chaperone for the outing while their mom and Uncle Hoyt worked in the field. It seemed like a good idea when our dream was invincible, but it didn't seem like such a great idea now. I reluctantly packed our beach bag, buckled the kids into their car seats, pulled out of our lane, and headed for the lake. Maybe a day of sunshine with Alex and Wyatt would do me good.

Once we arrived at the lake and the kids ran into the water, I sat down, buried my feet in the sand, and took a breath. When I looked around, I realized I was surrounded by happy families—babies, toddlers, moms, dads, and kids of all ages. As I took it all in, the reality dawned on me that this would never be my life. I would never pack a beach bag with water wings and tiny swimsuits, lather my kids in sunscreen, strap them in the truck, and spend a beautiful summer day at the lake making precious memories.

As that reality dawned, so did another: I had to go. I was not prepared for a day at the lake.

Neither was I ready for the small talk and questions in the parking lot on my escape to the safety of my vehicle.

"I didn't know you had kids!"

"You're right; I don't have kids. These are just on loan, and I have to return them."

I drove home in a zombie-like state. It was too painful to be present in the real world. I did not have the energy to answer Alex's questions about why her day in the sun had been cut so short.

I would learn in the coming days to listen to my body. Some days I needed to scrub floors, sweep out the shop, and reorganize my closet. On other days, I needed to lay in bed with the covers over my head because my emotions felt too intensely painful to manage outside of my blankets. Regardless of the kind of day I was having, I needed Hoyt close by. I didn't leave his side. I couldn't. He was the air I needed to breathe. I fell apart without him there beside me. I felt anxious and panicky. If I was alone, the demons I had buried in the dark corners of my heart came alive. I couldn't tame them by myself. I couldn't seem to function without Hoyt's reassuring presence. He was my anchor in the turmoil of my emotion. That meant if he was haying, I was riding in the little seat beside him. If he went to the city for parts for the tractor, I went too. If he got sick of me, he never said so.

Maybe he needed me, too.

Chapter 15

I am a reader, I always have been. For me, books have the power to transport me to another time and place, open my mind to new possibilities, transform my thinking, and ignite my creativity. Reading allows me to escape reality for a few precious hours. I was very prone to ear infections when I was a little girl. They were excruciatingly painful. When I was sick, my mom would give me Tylenol and a heating pad for my ear and would tuck me into my warm, cozy bed in my little pink room. She would read to me to take my mind off the pain. She read classics like *Anne of Green Gables* and *Little House on the Prairie*. I loved listening to Mom read. It was so comforting.

When infertility became my diagnosis, I naturally headed to the book store to find solace in a book. I wanted something to soothe my soul and calm my fears. I searched shop after shop and always came out empty-handed and disappointed.

The only books I could find were cure-all volumes full of suggestions on foods to eat to increase my chances of conception and foods to avoid to cure my infertility—as if it were something I could control and fix with a quick trip the grocery store. It made me feel shame—if only I had eaten a little less of this or a little more of that, my reproductive system would repair itself and I could have a child.

It seemed simple—and too good to be true.

My reading led to a string of wacky diets that I cajoled my beef-loving husband into following with me. He was a good sport and signed up for whatever whim I had embraced that particular week. One year, just before school started in the fall, I decided a green juice diet would lead us to health and happiness. You know the kind. I ground up spinach leaves, cucumbers, kale, and apples. If it was green, it went in the blender, topped off with a sprinkle of chia seeds. I could feel us getting healthier with every thick, green, goopy sip. We cut out sugar, gluten, caffeine, and pop.

One week into the diet, I decided to go to my school to spend a few hours working in my classroom. Hoyt came along to run errands while I prepared my lessons for the week. When he picked me up a few hours later, I asked what he felt like eating for supper. Hoyt confessed he wasn't hungry. When I demanded to know why—because my green juice had long since worn off and I was ravenous—he sheepishly admitted the green juice wasn't cutting it and so he had gone through the drive-thru for a burger. So much for solidarity. I lasted a few days longer until a colleague brought homemade fudge into the staff room to share. Soon my green juice diet was out the window and I was indulging in my second piece of fudge—without having cured my infertility.

My next cure-all was bone broth. During one of my many Google searches for at-home infertility cures, I read that bone broth could heal anything and everything that ailed you. We raise cattle and usually save one animal every year to fill our freezer with meat. The butcher always asks if we want the soup bones, which we always do. We save these bags of bones for our dog, Riley, as a special treat. He loves to chew on them. I immediately thought of the bags of frozen soup bones in my freezer. I excitedly announced to Hoyt that we were sitting on a gold mine. No wonder Riley was healthy; he had been eating these healing bones for years.

I grabbed a bag of soup bones from the freezer and placed them in the slow cooker to simmer. I added apple cider vinegar and a dash of turmeric, and we were ready to cure my infertility and my father-in-law's sore hip. I clipped on the lid and pressed start, eager to get my attempt at alchemy on the go, turning these simple soup bones into a rejuvenating elixir.

The bones bubbled merrily on my kitchen counter for two days, releasing their healing properties. I waited impatiently, ready to drink as much of the broth as quickly as I could in order to soak in all the health benefits contained in the brew. Finally, it was ready. I inhaled the fragrant steam as I lifted back the lid. I ladled a steaming scoop of this oily, yellow liquid into a bowl, eyeing it cautiously as I took a sip. I must have misread the recipe because although the broth was aromatic, it tasted vile and disgusting. I could not and would not eat the consommé, even if it would cure me.

Hoyt gave me his *I told you so look* as I poured my bowl of broth down the drain and prepared to give the rest of the batch to Riley—who thoroughly enjoyed his treat. It didn't appear as though bone broth was the answer to my infertility either.

My Google searches for infertility cures didn't end there. After my disappointing batch of bone broth, I decided to keep looking for another natural remedy. One of my infertility "eat this, not that" books listed beets as a food to eat for women who suffer from uterine fibroids. Apparently, there is a nutrient in beets rumored to slow the growth of the tumors and I was going to give it a try.

I like beets. I went beet crazy. Roasted beets, pickled beets, beet salad, cold beets, and hot beets. I was desperate to gain some semblance of control over my reproductive system. Eating beets was something that I could control and it gave me a sense of progress—as if I was moving closer and closer to my goal of motherhood with each purple forkful.

The end of my beet diet came one cold winter morning while I was whipping up a beet smoothie for breakfast. I must not have left the beets in the blender long enough because there were little chunks of beet in every sip. It looked like blood, tasted like dirt, and the pieces made me gag. That was the end of my love affair with beets. I would have to find another way to cure my infertility.

After the beet smoothie experience and my extensive reading about natural cures for infertility, I began to reflect and wonder. Yes, a balanced diet is essential to a healthy reproductive system and body, but why did I feel the need to go to such extremes? What made me feel so ashamed and guilty that I would agonize over which foods to eat and which to avoid no matter how disgusting the concoction or how deprived I felt? What caused me to feel like such a failure as a woman and as a wife that I was willing to try any solution no matter how absurd to fix my defective womb? I was desperate to gain control of my health and my ability to conceive. I bought into the cultural ideal that women should be mothers. As antiquated as that thinking might be, I was desperate to find my value as a woman. I was willing to go to any lengths to avoid childlessness.

The fact that I could find no inspirational books telling me not to worry and I would be okay in spite of my childlessness, upset me. I could not find any books in my local library or book store written by women highlighting another way, a different life, or the possibility of a fulfilling life after infertility. I felt as though the mindset around infertility seemed to be centered on "never give up, keep going at all costs, your value is found in motherhood." There didn't seem to be any other narrative or option for a purposeful life besides motherhood.

It was a suffocating thought.

That morning, standing over my kitchen sink, beet smoothie in hand, I wished for some calm voice of reason. I secretly longed to hear another woman tell me that it would be all right if I walked away from fertility treatments. The quiet voice of my intuition whispered the possibility of meaning beyond motherhood, sending goosebumps down my spine. I shook myself in the dark shadow of the early winter morning, willing that quiet voice—so contrary to my ingrained narrative of motherhood—to leave. I silenced my inner voice, unwilling to hear its message, and dumped my smoothie down the drain. I was not yet ready to give up on my dream of becoming a mother.

Chapter 16

I work at a small, community school. Our students are often children affected by poverty and addictions. I have seen parents who mistreat and neglect their children, show little affection, are disengaged from their child's lives—but are very fertile. I have seen parents who can't tear their eyes away from their cell phones to talk to their child, take them to the park, or read them a bedtime story—but are very fertile. I have seen parents who say they can't afford nutritious food or new shoes, can somehow afford drugs, alcohol, and cigarettes—but are very fertile. I have seen parents who are in and out of jail, use their children for gang-related tasks—but are very fertile. I have heard fertile parents tell me not to worry about my infertility because kids are a "pain in the ass anyway."

The abundant fertility of these parents seemed unjust to me. It added sting to my grief and made me angry because I know that Hoyt and I would've been wonderful parents. I felt cheated that we'll never have the opportunity to truly know who we would've been as parents. It seemed unfair that people who were far less able to provide for their children were blessed with babies and we were not. I deserved to have a child as much as anyone else.

I was meant to be a mother, too.

My mothering instinct and my nurturing spirit are hardwired. Teaching gives me an avenue to express those traits that feel so natural. I work with vulnerable children—boys and girls who don't have an adult in their corner, advocating for them and lighting up when they enter the room. I arrive at school every morning, determined to make the day a bit happier and safer for these children. I find myself often tempted to become overly invested in my students—beyond the call of duty. I worry if a particular child is fed and tucked up safe in bed at night. I bring warm mittens from home when I know a student has lost theirs. Secret stashes of treats are always hidden away in my desk to bring a smile to a sad face.

Supporting children in my teaching role is not the same as being a mother and nurturing my own children. While smiles, treats, and warm mittens bring me a sense of fulfillment, they do little to fill the place in my heart that is prepared and waiting for my own child who will never come.

One day a colleague found out I was childless. She commented that it was "just fine" that I had no children. Exasperated, I asked her to give me more information about how my heartache could be "fine." She elaborated that I was a "mother to many," meaning I worked with children at our school every day, and surely that would be enough to fulfill my biological urge for motherhood. The irony is not lost on me that I go to work each day and am invested in the success and well-being of other people's children, that I lay awake at night worrying about their safety, happiness, and basic needs, yet I cannot have my own children. Teaching allows me to show myself—and the world—that I would've been a good mom— as if my mother-worthiness was something that I needed to prove in order to gain more value as a woman in our society.

Another comment that I have received from parents and colleagues is that, "If you had children, maybe you would stop teaching, and kids who need your help would not receive it." I can't accept this reason for my infertility either. If I weren't at school doing my job, some other highly qualified and eager teacher would be. I am replaceable, and it is a job, only one part of my life. Although I do help children, teach them, and advocate for them, it's not up to me alone to ensure their well-being—that is primarily their parents' job.

My heart is big and loves easily. I have become invested in many children through my years of teaching, but teaching a child for one year and having a teacher-student relationship could never replace the love I would have for my own children, the bond I long for, or the sense of pride and wonder having a biological child would bring. Being a "mother to many" will never fill my longing to be a mother to one special child—my child.

Chapter 17

Throughout my years of fertility treatments and especially after my failed IVF cycle, I banned and boycotted everything baby related. I refused to go to baby showers or first birthday parties. I would not buy children's gifts or go into stores that sold baby-related merchandise. The sight of tiny shoes, beautiful cribs, and all the mandatory baby paraphernalia triggered my jealousy. I intentionally planned my grocery store route to avoid the baby supply aisle. The smell of baby powder and the boxes of diapers elicited my grief. I would only eat at restaurants that had a lounge because I couldn't bear to watch happy families eating together. The sound of babies crying and kids running around was like nails on the chalkboard of my heart. I avoided Walmart at all costs because whenever I forced myself to go, it appeared that every pregnant woman, frazzled mother, and happy family would also be needing toilet paper and cereal just like me. Social media was off limits because it seemed that the only thing that popped up on my news feed was expectant parents, birth announcements, maternity photos, gender reveals, top twenty baby name lists, and pictures of first birthdays.

At the end of the school day, parents often brought their babies and toddlers into the school to pick up their older siblings from my classroom. When a parent brought their bundle of joy into the building, my colleagues would be elated and coo happily to the baby. I, on the other hand, did not share in their eagerness to fuss over the child. The sight of a newborn held lovingly in its mother's arms brought instant tears to my eyes because my own arms were so obviously empty. I had to leave more than one parent meeting because the mother had brought her infant with her and I could not bear to be in the same room. Similar experiences happened at home. I had to mute the TV and run to my bedroom or hide my eyes in a blanket when one particularly heartwarming coffee commercial starring, you guessed it, babies, came on. It made me cry every time.

Catching glimpses of motherhood scared me because I saw first-hand the experience which I was missing. I felt resentful and afraid that it would never be our turn. I panicked to think Hoyt and I would never experience what it was like to wait nine months for a baby to arrive, to pick out a perfect name, or to bring a baby home from the hospital.

We watched from a distance as family and friends announced pregnancies and births. I yearned to know what it would be like to hold my own blond-haired, green-eyed child and to share my joy over our new baby. Each memory we watched other families make together—each Christmas morning, each special outing or activity, each milestone—was a token of a life I would never know. As these important events arose in our families, I wore a brave face and attended with a pasted-on smile, hopeful that no one would guess my secret sorrow.

Glimpses of motherhood forced me to confront my fear of childlessness—a reality I desperately wished to avoid. I feared that without the title of "mother," my life would be meaningless. Becoming a mother—and later a grandmother—seemed to be the ultimate goal of a woman's life. I had been conditioned to believe in that goal from the time I was a young girl, playing with my doll. To fall short of that ideal felt terrifying. I knew the progression of a life with children. Pregnancy, birth, first birthday, terrible twos, first day of school, driver's license, graduation—the life of parenthood followed a predictable pattern. There was no obvious pattern to childlessness. I had no idea how to navigate that life and I prayed I wouldn't have to find out.

I stopped attending occasions such as baby showers and first birthdays because these events left me in a constant state of comparison. Jealous feelings consumed my thoughts as I compared my childlessness with other women's fertility. I neglected and ignored the blessings in my life because I felt as though they were insignificant when compared to giving birth to a child and raising a family. A family of two is still a family—a fact that I overlooked because I was too caught up in comparison. My comparison of fertility versus infertility left me feeling bitter, jealous, and worthless.

While I reluctantly admit to having these emotions, I most certainly wished joy and happiness upon our family and friends. I am genuinely thankful when another woman experiences the miracle of birth because I know the science, the wonder, and the precision that is required to bring a child into the world. I feel relief to know that another woman does not have to know the pain and grief of infertility.

I didn't want my negative emotions to take joy from a friend or loved one during a special time like a baby shower. I didn't want to sour their experience or cause them pain. So, for a time, I chose to avoid these uncomfortable events because I could not attend and be truly happy for the occasion. I felt my sorrow casting a shadow on the moment. Babies are innocent and so perfectly precious. I couldn't allow myself to bring one ounce of sadness into their world that was only just beginning. Instead, I stayed at home, praying that our baby rollercoaster ride would soon be over and that I, too, could delight in motherhood.

Chapter 18

My sister, Rhonda, is petite and blonde. She has a quirky personality and a free spirit that she's not afraid to follow. She pushes the limits and challenges herself to be the best she can be and to find a path in life that is authentic and brings her joy.

Growing up, I was quiet, reserved, and thrived on routine and predictability—a rule-follower through and through. Rhonda sang jingles and danced in our living room—she was spirited, vibrant, and made her own rules. We had a typical sister relationship. We fought over clothes and stolen lip gloss, but deep down, loved each other fiercely.

When we were young, our contrasting personalities could, at times, cause friction. As we aged, we realized that we needed each other. Rhonda helps me to see the lighter side of life and to think outside of the traditional box. I keep Rhonda grounded. The bottom line is we love each other and would do anything for one another. Our lives were often in different stages and places because of our age difference, and our relationship—although strong and loving—would become distant, then closer, then distant again, as we lived our very different lives.

When Rhonda became engaged, we found ourselves working in the same city for the first time. Our proximity led to lunch dates and after work coffees and our bond strengthened with each passing day. We grew to know each other as adults, as women, not just sisters.

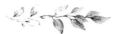

From the time I was four years old, I was confident that I would be a teacher when I grew up. There was no other profession that called to me the way teaching did. When I was in elementary school, I idolized my teachers. I watched them intently and then refined my own teaching skills, practicing with Rhonda in my basement where I had designed a makeshift classroom.

When Rhonda was five and I was thirteen, I set up a top-notch summer school in our basement with the intention of teaching my baby sister to read. Unfortunately, Rhonda was not a willing participant. She had other plans and none of them included sitting in a damp and musty basement learning the alphabet and printing her name.

At the time, I thought teaching meant high heels, coffee cups, Christmas concerts, and a bold lip color. I would find out early in my career that teaching is a hard and often thankless job. It is difficult to chase after Kindergarten students in high heels, coffee makes me jittery, and I prefer a shimmery lip gloss to a bold lipstick. I love teaching though, and if I had to choose a career again, I would choose education every time. My four-year-old self knew what she was doing.

Rhonda, on the other hand, was a tomboy who loved to play in the dirt and run around outside. She made up languages and thought she could communicate with our farm cats. She loved string and I would often come home from school to find the bedroom we shared tied up from bedpost to doorknob, closet door to dresser. No, she definitely was not interested in sitting on a hard chair for hours while I honed my teaching skills.

Rhonda's sense of adventure abounded. I owned a pink, lace-covered jewelry box that housed a ballerina who would spin around, dancing to the wind-up music when you opened the lid. I kept all my treasures in this jewelry box, including one-size-fits-all rings from birthday party treat bags and other jewelry I had been given that was more valuable. One day, my adventurous little sister took my jewelry box to use on her pirate's quest for jewels. Rhonda-the-pirate dug a hole in our garden, innocently dumped my treasures into the hole, and covered them with dirt. New to pirate life, she forgot to make a map and mark it with an X because when I returned home from school and realized my pink box was missing, she couldn't remember where she had buried the treasure. It may have been a rookie mistake on her part, but I kept my things under lock and key after that unfortunate incident.

My sister did not have such a conviction when it came to choosing a career path. I would tease her about her indecisiveness and ever-changing options. One month, she was going to be an artist, the next, a chef, and the month after that she wanted to become a yoga teacher on a beach in Mexico. The world was her oyster, the possibilities endless. I envied her free spirit. I was more a by-the-book, traditionalist. I thrive on repetition and certainty—and a career with a consistent paycheck.

In time, Rhonda would find her way and devote her life to caring for animals as a veterinary technician. Maybe she could communicate with those farm cats after all. Her love of animals meant a house full of pets, including rabbits, dogs, and a string of cats, some of whom were fosters from the humane society. If there was a stray cat nearby, it did not need to worry, because it was going home with Rhonda. She has a heart of gold and cannot stand to see anyone, human or animal, hurting or needing comfort.

From the time I was eight, Rhonda and I shared a bedroom. I remember arguing with my parents that it was not fair that I had to share a room; I was older, and I needed space and privacy. Rhonda's Winnie-the-Pooh posters were taking valuable wall space away from my Leonardo DiCaprio photographs. I was frustrated with having to share my space. I felt so much more mature and worldly, as teenage girls often do. It wasn't always like that, though.

Sweet memories were made in our little pink bedroom. When she was old enough, Rhonda would climb out of her crib and crawl in bed with me, and we would snuggle warmly together through the night. My mom would come into our room in the morning and find Rhonda in my bed more often than she would find her in the crib. Eventually, Mom took the mattress out of the crib and put it on the floor beside my bed where Rhonda would sleep contentedly, safe and sound, beside me—much the way my doll, Gail, had done, years earlier.

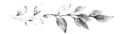

I may have offered comfort and safety to my sister when she was a little girl, but when I was at my lowest point as an adult, my sister would comfort me, be strong for me, and give me hope.

I left home when I was eighteen to attend university. When I went, Rhonda was only ten years old, still a child. I had been there for her first decade of milestones, but I would miss sharing the experiences that would provide the depth of character that this intelligent, poised, and determined young woman possessed—and so for a long time I held the image of her in my head as a little girl.

During my university years, my dad was in the fight of his life battling cancer. My mom was his advocate, nurse, caretaker, and companion. Rhonda was left at home to be brave for my parents and to live through the trauma and fear cancer leaves in its wake. Rhonda did not remember what life was like when Dad was healthy and Mom was not stressed and worried all the time.

The mood in my parent's house was one of thinly veiled hope with fear and anxiety lurking just below the surface. Cancer controlled our lives. Cancer decided the foods my parents ate and kept in the house because the chemotherapy drugs had left my dad's mouth raw and sore and his tastes skewed. He could tolerate only certain soft foods and the smell of some foods made him nauseous. The thermostat in my parent's home fluctuated to meet Dad's changing body temperature—shivering one moment, sweating the next.

When I came to visit, I walked on egg shells, afraid to speak too loudly or close a door with more force than intended as to not wake Dad up in case he was sleeping or had a headache. We all avoided anyone who had the slightest cough and made sure to keep our annual flu shot up to date—all in the attempt to protect my dad's immune system and keep him healthy. It was a traumatic time in all our lives, but especially for Rhonda. I believe caring for our Dad and being at home when he was suffering instilled a sense of compassion, empathy, and deep, deep love in my quirky, bubbly, free-spirited sister.

My brother and I would often think of Rhonda as our "little" sister since she never seemed to grow up in our eyes. We both felt a need to shelter her from the hard things the world would send our way. We did this subconsciously because we loved her and had been conditioned to protect her. Dad set the example when it came to his "little girl." We worked hard growing up. One of our yearly summer jobs was to rogue eighty acres of registered crop. To rogue meant walking arm length to arm length through a field of flowering mustard plants under the sweltering July sun, plagued by mosquitoes and allergies, looking for defective or inferior plants that were not supposed to be in the field. Once harvested, the seed gathered from the field would be sold to companies who would then distribute it to other farmers—all at a premium cost. Rouging was not a glamorous job, but it needed to be done. It instilled in us the value of hard work.

However, when Rhonda would complain it was too hot, or she had a headache, Dad would let her wait in the car where she took pictures of herself and the scenery with her toy camera while Derek and I walked the field—much to my brother's and my dismay. Dad would tell us, "She's just little, you know." We would grimace, we had heard the excuse before. We shrugged our shoulders and continued on. These incidences firmed up our belief that Rhonda was the "little" one and needed to be shielded.

Growing up, we watched my dad go through surgeries, use experimental chemotherapy drugs, attend countless medical appointments, and endure numerous procedures. We always knew that death was a possibility, but somehow, Dad always seemed to pull through—his life extended.

When my parents returned home early from a tropical vacation because Dad was unwell, we were anxious. Soon, it became apparent that he was very sick. His belly was oddly distended and he was in and out of hospital as his doctors tried valiantly to slow the spread of his cancer and relieve his symptoms. We took turns sitting with Dad in his hospital room, chatting and reminiscing about our most special memories. Dad shared life lessons and gave directions for what needed to be finished on his latest mechanical project and reminders to take care of our mom. He must've known his time was growing short—even if we were unwilling to accept that thought.

My phone rang in the middle of the night, jarring me awake. I had been sleeping deeply and awoke disoriented. As I searched in the dark for my phone, a feeling of dread and panic slowly spread through me. My brother was on the other end of the line when I answered.

"Something is really wrong, Jan. The paramedics think Dad had a stroke. He's in the ambulance now, Mom is riding with him to the hospital. Ashley and I will follow behind. Can you meet us there? The paramedics said I should call any family to come to say good bye. They don't think he has long. Hurry." My brother spoke in short and efficient sentences. He was calm, but I could feel the apprehension and fear in his voice coming through the phone.

I rushed to dress and Hoyt and I raced to the hospital. We had time to say our goodbyes, but still, Dad's death shocked us.

After the busyness of the funeral subsided, our grief slowly turned to numbness as we each tried to process our emotions in the void left behind.

My dad was a soft-spoken man with a kind heart and an ingenuity and work ethic only a prairie boy could have. He was always full of ideas and advice culled from experiencing life fully. For the first few years after he died, when life had thrown me a curveball or I was worried or unsure what to do, he would visit me in a dream. It was not my imagination conjuring up an image; I would wake and feel as though he had been right there with me. I could see him clearly and could hear his voice as he gave me advice that always started in the same way, "Well, you see, it's like this Jan...." Yes, I did see. I would feel immeasurably better, knowing what to do, until I became fully awake and realized that although the advice and comfort may have felt real, Dad was not there with me.

In the months after my dad's death, when something would go wrong, something upsetting happened, or hard decisions had to be made, my brother and I would talk it over, deciding together what to do and how to handle the situation. Sometimes Dad would come to me in a dream comforting me with his usual wisdom.

Mom was deep in her grief so Derek and I tried to protect her from more pain, just as we tried to protect Rhonda. We comforted each other as best we could, but most definitely kept whatever decision that had to be made or whatever problem had arisen to ourselves. It was an unspoken understanding that we would not tell Rhonda because we did not want to cause her any more pain or sorrow. Nothing should steal her joy or cause her to worry and it was up to us to make sure she was safe and content.

We had underestimated the strength and tenacity of our spirited sister. She was no longer a child; she was a grown woman and no longer needed us to protect her. She could look after herself just fine. Rhonda did not appreciate our underestimation of her strength of character and nor did she appreciate being left out of discussions and decision making. She would often say in frustration, "You guys don't tell me anything!" She was right; we didn't, but our instinct was to protect. Our intentions were good.

When our miracle baby did not appear, my dad didn't visit me in my dreams despite the intense emotional pain I was experiencing. How could that be? I needed him. Initially, I had felt so sure about our IVF cycle ending with a pregnancy partly because I believed my dad would send me a baby from Heaven. Partly because I believed that the smooth, pink apple on my previously barren tree was a sign of fertility sent to me from God. I was disappointed to think that my dad would let me down. Surely there were lots of babies in Heaven; they could spare one for me. The thought of my dad taking care of my children until I could do so was comforting. Maybe he still is taking care of my babies until I get to Heaven to take over.

Chapter 19

Before our first round of IVF had begun, Hoyt and I decided to tell our family and close friends about our plans. I couldn't contain our secret. I thought I might burst if I didn't tell someone. I felt ready to share our excitement and was delighted in telling our news. When my IVF failed, I realized this might not have been the best plan because then I had to call and tell everyone, answer their questions, and listen to their advice and attempts at comfort. When I shared my disappointment with Rhonda, she sympathized with me.

Then the subject was closed.

In the following weeks and months, the shadow of my infertility awkwardly filled the pauses and quiet moments during my conversations with Rhonda. It was always there, but we never openly discussed it. I wanted to shield my sister from my pain and did not want to lay my burden on her shoulders. It was my instinct to protect Rhonda—even if it meant keeping my sorrow a secret. When we were together, I pasted on a smile and pretended to be "fine."

As the months wore on, Hoyt and I both started to heal, and our sorrow lessened. We became restless—because something always felt like it was missing. We were not complete, there was a void in our lives. That restless feeling was caused by the empty place in our hearts reserved for our child, the one who we waited for but who never came.

Time had started to heal our hurt and we began to talk again about our desire to be parents. We were not ready to give up yet, even after all we had suffered. Slowly, cautiously, we started to wonder, could we try again, were we strong enough to hope again, was there another way? We discussed our options, few as they were, and what path we could take if we wanted to walk any at all.

Our biggest problem was that my ovaries were covered with scar tissue and were so damaged they no longer could function properly to produce eggs. That hurdle could be overcome in one of three ways. We could try fertility drugs at an extremely high dosage with the hope that my ovaries would respond—which would cost a fortune. We could purchase eggs from the United States—which would cost a fortune. Or we could find someone willing to donate eggs for us to use—which would also cost a small fortune. We discussed our options and our finances at length and came up with no satisfactory solution.

Childlessness, however, was not a great option either.

We would talk, wonder, research, and change our minds continuously as we tried to sort out what we should do. We could agree that regardless of which option we chose, it would be expensive. We decided that if the process could result in a child, regardless of cost, it would be worth it. Our child would be worth it. We rationalized that children were costly for any couple regardless of how their child was conceived; we just had to start paying for ours earlier than most couples. We were logical and tried to rationalize the cost into something we could accept as reasonable, even if our bank account hovered dangerously near the red and our credit cards were nearly over the limit—not yet replenished after our previous IVF cycle. Even though we both agreed that we were committed to building our family, the looming expenses felt ominous.

I felt with certainty that trying fertility drugs and IVF again was not the way for us. I worried my body would once again betray me. I dreaded the thought of the pain of procedures, the tests, the trips to the city, and the needles. My pulse quickened at the thought of the money we would spend—and potentially waste— on fertility drugs only to be left with maxed-out credit cards and utter disappointment. I had spent the better part of the past year rebuilding my life and I was resigned to move on, childless. I was terrified that if we tried again and the treatments failed, I would once again be devastated, but this time, I worried I would not be strong enough to recover. Another round of IVF was out of the question for me. Hoyt agreed. As much as I longed for a child that was biologically mine, I knew another round of fertility treatments was not the answer, so we kept searching, trying to find our way.

Our second option was to purchase eggs. It was a possibility, but we wondered at what cost. We did not know if we were comfortable choosing a donor and raising a stranger's child. Would I bond with a child I carried but who was not biologically mine? How would we explain our decisions to our child, how would our families react to this unconventional attempt at parenthood? We still clung to the fantasy of having our biological child. We kept this option of purchasing eggs on the table but kept searching for answers, not quite sure this option was the right one.

Putting IVF and purchasing eggs as possible solutions aside, left us with one last option. We could find a woman who would be willing to donate her eggs for us to use.

Hoyt and I discussed our options. The prospect of finding someone generous enough to donate her eggs for us to use seemed preposterous. Who could we possibly ask to do this enormous and selfless act of kindness? It was something I didn't feel like I could ever ask of anyone. It was too much.

With some research, we learned that if we chose to take this route, the process would require our donor to begin a regimen of fertility drugs to grow her eggs. The eggs would be retrieved, fertilized in a lab with a donation from Hoyt, allowed to develop to a viable stage, and then transferred to my waiting uterus. Meanwhile, I would also begin a round of fertility drugs that would simultaneously suppress my ovaries and prepare my uterus for implantation of our embryos. This option would require all the tests, medications, needles, and trips to the city I was trying so hard to avoid.

Nevertheless, we reasoned that if we were to find a woman willing to donate her eggs, at least we would know that person and their history. It wasn't quite as scary as choosing an unknown donor. We rationalized that if we could find someone who was young and healthy and responded well to the fertility drugs, we could potentially have a number of viable, healthy eggs that we could fertilize and freeze so we would have a bank for the future— eggs we expected to use for our multiple future children. We agreed this seemed to be our best option.

"Why don't you ask your sister if she'd help us," Hoyt suggested one evening as I ladled rich, spicy meat sauce onto the spaghetti on my plate. "She would be the perfect person to donate eggs. I bet she'd do it. What do you think?" he continued, around bites of pasta.

Months earlier, during a conversation with Rhonda, I had casually mentioned the possibility of egg donation. My sister had offered to donate her eggs but I had quickly dismissed the idea because I felt like it was too much to ask.

We listed every woman we knew and talked about the pros and cons of asking each person our outrageous favor, but we kept circling back to one person: Rhonda, my sister.

For Hoyt, the argument was simple. If Rhonda donated her eggs for us, our child would have DNA almost identical to mine. It would be as close as we could get to our biological child. If Rhonda donated her eggs, we would know that our child would be at risk for cancer and diabetes due to family medical history and would likely need an inhaler, thanks to Hoyt's asthma, but we could protect our child from these medical conditions and try to prevent them. Hoyt rationalized it would be just like having my own child, except this child would be shorter and blonder than me.

I disagreed. Strongly.

It was my job to protect my sister, shield her from the difficult parts of life. I could not, in any universe, in any space or time, ever, under any uncertain terms, ask my sister to do this outrageous thing for me. I cringed at the thought of dragging her into the middle of my infertility nightmare.

Ultimately, we could not move on.

Our discussion in the kitchen that evening kept turning back to Rhonda, as our dinner cooled on our plates. The thought of asking my sister to donate her eggs made me uncomfortable. I would be carrying my husband's and my sister's child and raising it as my own. Technically, I would be the auntie, and she would be the mom, except it would be the opposite. How would we explain their origins and the family dynamic to our child? How would we answer the inevitable questions? What if we unintentionally damaged our child emotionally with their unconventional conception? What if the community found out and our child suffered the consequences of an unforgiving and uneducated public?

I worried, if we did this, what would happen when the baby grew into a teenager and said those infamous words only teenagers can say: "I don't have to listen to you, you are not my mom!" The child would be right. I wouldn't be their mom, technically speaking, so why would they have to listen to me? What if Rhonda and I grew apart a few years down the road and she wanted her baby back? What would our families think? Worse, what would they say? How would Rhonda's partner, Kyle, feel about egg donation?

My biggest fear, however, was that if we did ask Rhonda for her eggs, and she agreed, if we went through the process, but it did not work, I would be devastated. This time it would not just be Hoyt and me who were invested and disappointed if the IVF or embryo transfer failed. Rhonda and Kyle would be affected, too. I did not want to knowingly put my sister or Kyle in a position that had tremendous potential to end in hurt.

Our spaghetti was cold and congealed—long forgotten during the intensity of our conversation that night. The late news was coming on and it was time for bed. We had too many questions and not enough answers for one night. We would bring this scenario up occasionally in wistful conversation over the next few weeks, each of us contemplating the repercussions and the possibilities of egg donation during the private moments of our day and sharing them when we were alone and free to hypothesize, question, and wonder. Slowly, I started to feel more comfortable with the idea of egg donation.

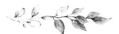

One weeknight, I arrived home from work later than usual. I was grumpy and hungry after a long day and so I was trying to make supper in a hurry. While I was pulling ingredients out of the fridge to prepare dinner, Hoyt raised the topic of egg donation once again. It was terrible timing, but we talked about it anyway. Soon my mood softened, my day melted away, and I could focus on this crucial conversation with my husband. The discussion had started similarly to so many previous conversations, us wondering but always seeming to have more questions than answers.

Frustrated, I said to Hoyt, "It isn't even worth talking about unless we know for sure whether Rhonda would even consider donating her eggs to us." I slammed cupboard doors and drawers as I moved around the kitchen, collecting pots and cooking utensils.

"Fair enough," he agreed. "So, are you going to call her or what?"

I wasn't ready for that. I had not prepared for it. I was just there in the kitchen, innocently making supper. I could not possibly make such a life changing phone call on a Tuesday night, could I? Besides, what would I even say, how could I ask, what if she said no and it made things awkward between us? Even scarier, what if she said yes?

Hoyt held the phone out to me, and reluctantly, I took it, dialing the familiar number with trepidation. Three rings and Rhonda answered, cheerful as always, unaware of the bombshell I was about to drop on her life. We exchanged the usual pleasantries about work and the weather, and then the conversation came to a standstill. My heart was beating too fast, and my mouth was dry.

Then Rhonda asked, "So, what did you need?"

Now was my chance, it was time to get on with it, say the words, ask the question, wait for an answer, and know for sure. I started strong but quickly lost my nerve.

"Well you see, we have a question for you, it is a big one, I hate to ask, you can say no if you want to, but we were wondering, if maybe, possibly, you'd consider ..."

Rhonda interrupted me in an exasperated tone. "For heaven's sake, Jan, what do you want to ask me? Just say it!"

It was too much, too close to my heart, the emotions too raw, and I started to cry. Through my tears, I finally asked the question. "We were wondering if you would consider donating eggs for us to use."

There. The words were out there hanging in the silence between us, Rhonda processing the request and its implications, me dreading her response. I could not take those words back or un-say them now; it was too late. All I could do was wait for her answer.

I did not have to wait long. My sweet sister asked, "Well, what would I have to do?"

We were off. The course was set, our baby rollercoaster was set into action. The conversation that followed was full of questions, which I tried my best to answer. I explained the process of an IVF cycle from my past experiences. We talked about the ins and outs of needles, timing, and fertility drugs. We talked about what sharing a child would look like and what it would mean to us. There were no more tears while we talked things over. We agreed Rhonda would take some time to think about making this sacrifice for us, talk it over with Kyle, and when they had come to a decision, she would let us know.

As I hung up the phone that night, I was filled with a deep, resounding love for my sister, her kindness, and her willingness to consider donating her eggs for me. It was overwhelming. Most of all, I once again had hope for a child, something I had been certain I would never feel again.

Hope is like a double-edged sword, bittersweet. At times, hope was be the only thing that kept me going. Hope was also the thing that could bring me to my knees at a moment's notice. I had been disappointed so often—my coaster car slamming down the track from the full height of hope too many times before. I was afraid to let myself feel encouraged or expectant. To hope felt too risky. Admitting that I wanted to try again for a child—especially in this unconventional way—exposed my true desires and made me feel vulnerable. If I didn't hope, didn't feel, didn't acknowledge, maybe, I told myself, I could avoid loss, disappointment, and sadness.

I knew these dark emotions too well. The ache in my bones still lingered from the previous trauma of loss and I wanted to avoid feeling those emotions again at all costs. The problem was, when I numbed the dark, I numbed the light as well. So, slowly, cautiously, I let a little light in the cracks of my heart, allowing myself to once more hope for a child.

Chapter 20

    I am terrible at keeping secrets. The people close to me quickly learn I shouldn't be trusted with keeping juicy news to myself for long. Of course, I know the difference between personal, sacred information that must remain confidential and the other details of life. The perfect gift that I've picked out for your birthday, who has a crush on who, what time your surprise party starts, where the Christmas gifts are hidden away—these are the secrets I have trouble keeping quiet. To know a secret is to feel like my chest is bursting and the secret is caught in my throat, just waiting to jump out the first chance it gets. I itch to tell the good news or to spread the joy because it's just too exciting not to share.

    Sometimes I make a conscious decision to share a secret. I rationalize that if I give someone a clue or if I casually drop hints into a conversation and that person makes a correct guess, then I haven't given the surprise away. Nor am I any longer responsible to keep the secret to myself. At other times, the secret bursts forth from my mouth, unannounced, before my brain can stop it, taking me by surprise. If you want something kept quiet, you might want to think twice before you tell me because your secret might not be secret for long.

When I was still young enough to believe in Santa Claus, but old enough to lead my brother astray, I had an unhealthy obsession with searching the nooks and crannies of our house to find Christmas gifts my mom had purchased and hidden away. The gifts were to stay concealed until my parents wrapped them on Christmas Eve and set under the tree in the wee hours of Christmas morning, but I couldn't wait to find out what my gifts would be.

One fateful afternoon in late December, my mom went to town for groceries and left Derek and me with my grandmother. When Mom was safely on her way to town, and Grandma was busy in the kitchen with soap operas blaring in the background, I enlisted the help of my trusting little brother, and the search began in earnest. My mom had underestimated my determination and skill at locating presents and I quickly found her stash. She had hidden our gifts in the same place she always did—in the back of her closet behind a trunk. I was no amateur—this hiding spot hadn't even posed a challenge for an expert like me.

We must have been well-behaved that year because my brother and I were ecstatic to find out that Santa was bringing us sleds. These sleds were not your average crazy carpet or toboggan—they were the Cadillac model, with comfortable seats, a racing stripe, two red hand brakes—and they were calling our names. Now that I knew these sleds were tucked away in my mother's closet, I couldn't simply go back to reading a book or playing with my doll. Mom was in town and would surely be there a while, and since Grandma was a softie who didn't ask questions, we decided it would be a real thrill if we tried out the sleds and then quickly returned them to their closet hiding spot before Mom returned home.

I imagined the sting on my cheeks as cold winter air rushed past, feeling as though I was flying down the hill. I could hear the crunch of powdery snow as my sled glided over the banks. My brother had a mischievous grin on his face and a familiar sparkle in his eye. He grabbed his sled and was lugging it out of our parents' bedroom before I could stop him. He was headed for the glistening hill that bordered our driveway. I knew I couldn't rest until I had tried a few runs with my new sled.

I picked up the red rope handle, "Wait for me!" I called after my brother, and hurried to catch up.

There were many holes in our strategy, but we were too young to recognize them. Even if we had, we would have ignored the weakness in our plan—we were eager to try out our new sleds and no one was going to stop us.

We managed to struggle into our winter clothes and sneak the sleds outside past our inattentive babysitter to the freedom of the steep, snowy ditch in front of our house. We hopped on our sleds and let them rip down the slippery hill, crashing to a stop at the bottom, leaving us laughing with glee in a heap of snow. We trudged back up the hill and whooshed down, again and again, enjoying every trip over the shimmering snow.

Suddenly, Mom was pulling into the lane, home from her grocery shopping trip. She did not look happy; we could tell that from a distance. We must have lost track of time and now we were in trouble, deep trouble. The names of two young sled stealers quickly moved to the naughty list, and Santa did not bring our sleds on Christmas morning, much to our disappointment—but not surprise.

I don't know what happened to our sleds—this is my only memory of them. My mom must've been thoroughly annoyed with Derek and me that day. She was unrelenting in our consequence and teaching us a valuable life lesson about snooping and stealing. The next time we stayed with our grandma, she was much more attentive. Maybe she learned a lesson that day as well.

You might think I would have learned my lesson about keeping secrets after an experience like that. I'm sure my parents were hoping I had, but sadly, I had not. The year I turned eighteen, my dad turned fifty. My mom had planned a surprise party for Dad and had shared her plans with me. One night at the supper table, Mom was talking about commitments on the calendar and upcoming appointments for the week.

I innocently asked, "Hey, Mom, isn't that the same day as Dad's surprise party?"

So much for my secret keeping skills. It was the story of my life—one poorly kept secret after another.

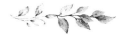

A week went by after our initial conversation with Rhonda. Hoyt and I waited anxiously each night for the call from my sister that would give us renewed hope, another chance at parenthood, and our ticket back onto the rollercoaster ride of emotions. Finally, my phone rang, and Rhonda's name appeared on the screen. I answered, anxious to hear from her but dreading her answer at the same time.

"Hello?" I answered on the second ring. We chatted for a few minutes and then the conversation came to a pause. I waited, breath caught in my chest while Hoyt stood anxiously by my side.

Rhonda broke the silence.

"I've thought a lot about donating eggs for you, Jan. Kyle and I have talked and debated about different scenarios and potential problems that could come up. We still have some questions about the procedures and some details about the legal side of egg donation but no matter what we talked about, or what problem we might foresee, Kyle and I both feel that the benefits outweigh the possible risks or problems. If I can do this for you, I want to. I will donate my eggs for you. When can we get started?" Rhonda asked exuberantly.

I was speechless. I was overwhelmed with emotion. Relief washed over me. I exhaled, releasing some of the fear, tension, and anxiety that I had been carrying silently hidden in the dark corners of my heart. Layers of emotions color that moment. Intense love for my sister, joy at the prospect of another chance for a child, potential liberation from childlessness, renewed hope, and excitement.

I was overwhelmed by the powerful emotions brought on by my sister's generosity. I tried—unsuccessfully—to put into words what this gift meant to me. I am still astonished when I think about the enormity of my sister's love and compassion; it is awe-inspiring. The wonder and excitement were palpable in our kitchen that evening.

"She said yes!" I shouted to Hoyt once I had ended the call. He wrapped me in his arms and we clung to each other, tears wet on our cheeks. I remember every detail of that phone conversation— where I was standing, the lighting in our kitchen, the sound of my heart beating in my chest, the way my breath caught in my throat, and the depth of emotion that I felt. Hoyt and I fell asleep that night, holding each other's hands and holding the hope of our child in our hearts.

The next morning, I made the call to our fertility clinic—the clinic I had vowed never to return to—and made an appointment to see Dr. Lucky Strike. Just before Christmas, Hoyt, Rhonda, and I found ourselves sitting in the doctor's office discussing IVF, the process of egg donation, fresh versus frozen embryo transfers, cost, what to expect, and the odds of successful egg donation.

Rhonda was young, healthy, and fertile. Dr. Lucky Strike predicted a good chance of retrieving healthy eggs, creating a bank of viable embryos to hold on reserve, and having a successful first pregnancy with multiple successful pregnancies in the future. Dr. Lucky Strike said all the right things in his office that afternoon. That was it. That was all it took. I was fully committed and tied in tight on the rollercoaster ride one more time. I had jumped back into the wild ride of fertility treatments in spite of my fears and worries—this time with my sister strapped in beside me.

I left the clinic that day, awash with relief. I could still achieve my dream of being a mother. Rhonda was going to give me this precious gift of life and it was going to work because the odds were in our favor. We were in this together. Success seemed to be the only possible destination for our trip around the rollercoaster track.

I forgot, unfortunately, that I had been on this ride before, more than once. I ignored the gnawing feeling of my intuition reminding me to be cautious with my hope and to guard my heart. I had forgotten the plummet into the dark, the free fall, the sudden stops, the crash, and the moments frozen in time.

Looking back on that day, I remember leaving the clinic giddy with excitement and confidence. I put my faith and my future into Dr. Lucky Strike's hands once again. I wished so badly to hear that I could have a baby that I disregarded the warning signs and my intuition telling me to be careful. Dr. Lucky Strike's lofty statements, his easy smile, and his eagerness to obtain my credit card number should have made me pause for a reality check. My intuition whispered questions in my heart. Would Rhonda—and would I—respond to the fertility drugs? Would my uterus support a pregnancy? Could we afford the procedures? Could my heart—or my marriage—survive if our plan failed?

I wanted to have a child and to be a mother—that goes without saying. If I was being totally honest with myself though, I am less sure if my urge to conceive outweighed my desperate urge to fulfill the assumption that all women should be mothers, to find my value and purpose as a woman in the role of motherhood, to give my husband a child to carry on his legacy, and to be a "good" wife. I was anxious to avoid a life of pitying looks from acquaintances who learn that I am childless. I was unwilling to admit that while my sister's egg donation was a fantastic opportunity—our best option—it was not a guarantee and it certainly wouldn't fix the unhealthy narrative about womanhood running on repeat through my brain.

Fertility is a business, and it preys on childless women when we are most vulnerable. Yes, fertility treatments were designed to assist women like me and some treatment cycles are successful. Make no mistake, however, fertility clinics are also about making money. I fell for the sales pitch and bought in hook, line, and sinker. Phrases like, *"let's make a baby"*, and *"multiple future pregnancies"* made me feel invincible. Failure was not on the table; I wouldn't even let it enter my mind. Hope is a fine line to straddle. You need hope, a positive attitude, and a cup-half-full mentality to survive this baby rollercoaster ride of emotions, but hope can also be a dangerous emotion that can leave you in agony within a split second.

Chapter 21

Our initial appointment with Dr. Lucky Strike was over, and our decision had been made. We chose to pursue egg donation and embryo transfer. The possibility of becoming parents outweighed our worries and concerns. The dates for the cycle had been selected and the first fees were paid. We agreed without discussion that this time we would not share our plans with anyone—not our parents, our siblings, or our friends. Our mission was top secret and most definitely under lock and key.

There is a difference between a secret and something private. A secret can be a happy and welcome surprise, or it can be a dark and ugly truth that can never be shared. Our decision to try for our sweet baby one more time was not a surprise, nor was it an ugly truth. This time, our decision just felt too private to share. During our first round of IVF, we told everyone and anyone who would listen. It was awful and embarrassing having to call and inform all those people there was no baby, no happy announcement. We didn't want to do that again.

This time, we decided to keep our decision quiet and private until we had the exciting news we hoped we could soon share. Then, if the IVF worked and I was pregnant, we would shout it from the rooftops, or at least with a tastefully done photoshoot. You know the kind—the ones with two pairs of big cowboy boots with a tiny pair in between them. For the first time in my life, it was easy for me to keep quiet about my struggle to become pregnant and about our upcoming fertility treatments; I didn't share with anyone. I tucked this sacred and private information away.

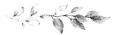

The next five months were busy for me. I purposely planned my life to be full of demanding tasks in order to keep myself from overthinking every aspect of our egg donation and embryo transfer which were scheduled for June. I focused on staying positive, keeping active, getting my weight in check, and optimizing my body for a baby—no more Cheezies and ice cream for me.

I had recently started a new job as a Student Support Teacher at my school, which meant I spent my days teaching children who struggled to learn to read. I worked with students from Kindergarten to Grade 8. I loved it. I'm passionate about teaching and I felt a huge sense of responsibility to be able to give my students the gift of learning to read—even if they were not as excited about the idea as I was.

I poured myself into my work and spent hours researching best practices, looking at data, and planning lessons for my students. In March, I registered for a university class to start my Certificate of Inclusive Education, a technical institute course to learn how to inseminate cattle artificially, and a conference to be held in beautiful Victoria, British Columbia about youth at risk and community schools. Of course, this was in addition to my full-time job, my duties as a rancher's wife, and the busyness of calving season. I didn't have time to worry or overthink anything.

My days were full and each night I fell blissfully asleep the moment my head hit the pillow.

The days flew by in a blur and soon it was the end of the school year. There is nothing like June in a non-air conditioned, 110-year-old elementary school. The kids are rambunctious, the teachers are tired, and everybody is ready to be done. The classrooms are sweltering and excitement fills the air—freedom is just around the corner.

This particular June was no exception, but for the first time in three years, I finished the school year without having to take a medical leave for surgery or bedrest. I was healthy, I was ready to dive into another round of fertility treatments, and it was our turn to become parents.

This cycle of IVF would prove to be very different from my previous experiences. This time we were not going through the unnerving process alone. We had Rhonda and Kyle to share with us the uncertainty, the excitement, and the miracle of our wild ride. Egg donation comes with a long list of hoops to jump through before the procedures can begin—some medical, some clerical, all difficult. Throughout each new challenge, we were able to find humor and laughter largely due to Kyle and his wicked sense of humor. Hoyt has a sense of humor too, and when Kyle and Hoyt joined forces, we often found ourselves laughing until tears were running down our faces and our bellies hurt. We were able to relax and find joy during this otherwise stressful time.

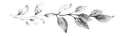

While I was excited at the prospect of motherhood in my future and grateful for my sister's generosity, I was also apprehensive. There were countless complicated, tedious, and often frustrating steps that had to be completed in sequence before we could start our egg donation process and before we could even begin to think about the actual medical procedures. Dealing with the legal, medical, and logistical specifics required next-level organizational precision. Dealing with the emotions and anxiety brought on by the all-too-familiar initial phase of our impending IVF cycle required courage and vulnerability. Courage to accept an unknown outcome and to commit to this unconventional path to motherhood. Vulnerability to allow ourselves to feel hopeful once more.

My past experiences with fertility treatments had not ended well. They had taught me that no matter how much I prepared or how bright the future looked, something inevitably could go wrong and my chances at being called "Mom" could once again slip through my fingers. I worried that at some point during the endless schedule of tests and appointments, something would happen, my broken reproductive system would take a stand against me, and we would hear, "Oops, sorry, we made a mistake, this isn't going to work out after all."

Imagine my surprise when each test came back normal, each appointment went well, and every stage of our treatments was right on schedule. Our rollercoaster car was inching its way up the track, gaining momentum with every breath I took. I could smile back at the secretary when I left the office, although I'm not sure she recognized me when I wasn't crying. With each normal result we received, I let myself become a little more hopeful, a little more certain, and envision a future that looked a little brighter.

At one appointment early in the consultation process, I was feeling anxious. My old fears and worries about my body's response to the drugs and its ability to support a pregnancy came to the surface once again. Dr. Lucky Strike smiled his too-big grin and assured me in his silky-smooth voice that just recently he had transferred embryos to a forty-six-year-old woman whose uterus was in much worse shape than mine, and she was currently pregnant with twins. I calmed down immediately and decided that if a woman in her forties with a bad uterus could have twins, I was confident that I would have no problem at all. What I failed to ask—and what Dr. Lucky Strike failed to mention—was how many rounds of IVF this woman had endured, how many thousands of dollars she had spent to achieve a successful pregnancy, whether her marriage had survived her fertility treatments, and what sacrifices she had made along the way.

Be careful, listen to your intuition, and ask questions. IVF fails more often than it succeeds. Each case is unique. Each woman is different. Allow yourself to hope, but don't let promises, false hopes, and so-called guarantees cloud your judgement or quiet your inner voice of wisdom. Was my doctor competent? Yes. Did he have my best interests at heart? Maybe, maybe not. Did he give me all the facts, the good and the bad, so I could decide based on something other than pure, raw emotion? Not exactly. Of course, it was my responsibility to search for the facts, to ask the questions, to be objective, and to make an informed decision, but it was also my doctor's responsibility to be honest, to avoid sugar coating and giving hope where there was none to give.

Then again, it is easy to hear only the things we want to hear.

Chapter 22

The first hoop for me was a mock trial. Dr. Lucky Strike needed to test my body to see if I would respond to the fertility drugs. These drugs would thicken the lining of my uterus to make a safe and cozy home for my babies to live in for nine months. It was just pills this time—no needles—much to my relief. I was nervous about the trial and kept putting it off. I was afraid it might reveal that my reproductive system didn't respond to the fertility drugs and I wouldn't be able to carry our babies after all. I thought next month I would be healthier, in six weeks I would lose even more weight, maybe I could begin the trial in two months when I would be in top "mom" condition. Eventually, my procrastination had to come to an end, and I forced myself to begin the round of drugs.

When the two-week-long trial was finished, I made an appointment with our clinic for an ultrasound to see whether my uterus lining had thickened the required amount. I was quiet on the trip to the city. I was trying to decide how I would react, how I would handle the news that my uterus had not responded, and what I would do then. I had convinced myself I would receive bad news because I felt like it was easier to expect and plan for disappointment than it was to be confident and hopeful only to be devastated by potentially negative results.

Apprehensively, Hoyt and I arrived at the clinic. We were met by Dr. Lucky Strike and I was taken away for an ultrasound exam while Hoyt waited in the reception area. I had been in the ultrasound room countless times before, and most of those times, I had received unwelcome news while my feet were in the stirrups.

Not this time.

I was amazed to see Dr. Lucky Strike smiling down at me from his end of the exam table. My uterus was normal, the lining had thickened, everything was fine, and we could proceed as planned. *Normal, fine, proceed as planned*—these weren't words I was accustomed to hearing from any doctor. Relief flooded through me.

I closed my eyes in a silent prayer of gratitude then hurried to dress behind the flimsy *Live, Love, Laugh* shower curtain in the change room and sought out Dr. Lucky Strike before we left. I wanted confirmation. Should he maybe double check my scans? Was he certain everything was fine? Was he positive my uterus looked normal? Was he sure he was looking at the right chart? Dr. Lucky Strike flashed me his easy smile and smoothly assured me that yes, everything was fine and we could go ahead with the donation and transfer. We could go home and relax. Rhonda was young and fertile, and I was normal. Everything was fine.

Next on our long list was to meet with a lawyer and draw up a contract for the egg donation. The agreement was a necessary part of the process that would protect everyone and would bring the grey areas a little closer to black and white. A handshake and a pinky promise wouldn't suffice in this case. Egg donation is cloaked in grey and has countless repercussions for everyone involved no matter how altruistic the intentions. I was only starting to grasp the enormity of what we were about to do. Talking to the lawyer forced us to consider scenarios and details we might've otherwise overlooked. We needed to make decisions like whose name would be listed as the mother of the child on the birth certificate, what would happen to any frozen embryos if Hoyt and I became divorced or one of us died, and who paid for coffee on our many trips to the city.

We had never discussed these details. We were naïve to the fact that they were details that we had to consider. But when you are creating a life with a donation such as this, no detail is too small, no scenario too scary, and no feeling is too sacred for discussion.

Our lawyer came highly recommended by our fertility clinic staff. So, we typed the address into our navigation system and set off to meet her. As we drove, the neighborhood became sketchier, older, and dirtier. Soon, we saw a pawnshop or payday loans office on every corner. The navigation system suddenly announced we had arrived at our destination and we saw a bright yellow and green building that looked more like a Caribbean hut than a law office. We thought that, surely, this had to be a mistake. To our amusement, it was, in fact, the lawyer's office, and it oddly shared the building with a pool hall. We went inside, met with the lawyer, and came out with a contract on which we could all agree. We set the document in the dark bottom of the console in our truck for safekeeping and carried on with our busy day.

Next on our to-do list was a psychological screening and evaluation. Rhonda, Hoyt, and I were each required to attend a session with a psychologist to ensure that we were mentally and emotionally stable prior to beginning the egg donation process. The purpose of the sessions was to discuss strategies to protect our mental health throughout the process and to make sure that we fully understood the ramifications of egg donation. It was also a time to speak honestly and freely about how we were feeling.

Seeing a psychologist was a new experience for me. Talking with mental health practitioners was not common in our family circle. We were proud of the fact that we took care of our own issues, we did not need nor want to talk to psychologists. If something happened, we just toughened up and carried on. There was no working through emotions or asking for advice. Even after my dad had passed away and none of us were handling it well, we never went to talk to a counselor, either individually or as a family. The thought never crossed our minds. In hindsight, I wish we had spoken to somebody during those tough times. Sometimes the things we go through and experience in life are bigger than we are and more than we can handle—no matter how strong or tough we think we may be.

Infertility is one of those things.

However, this time talking to a psychologist was mandatory. None of us knew what to expect. I had spent the time leading up to the appointment in a tumultuous emotional state. I worried I would cry during the interview or I would say the wrong thing and reveal the fragile hold I had on my emotions. I thought if I exposed too much or not enough of myself the doctor would decide I was unfit to be a parent or not stable enough to go through the process and we wouldn't be able to proceed. I was concerned that the psychologist would tap into the deep well of emotions and hurt that was my infertility. I was on edge during the entire two-hour drive to our appointment.

Hoyt expertly navigated through the busy city streets and we arrived at the office with plenty of time to spare. The sign on the door indicated we were at Dr. Phil's office. Of course, he was not Dr. Phil the TV host, but Dr. Phil, the psychologist who would decide if we would qualify as fit parents.

The receptionist called our names and led Hoyt and me back to the doctor's office. The room was dimly lit and filled with heavy, dark furniture and ornate decorative pieces. We settled comfortably onto the chocolate brown leather couch and let the low lighting and quiet atmosphere envelope us.

Within minutes of meeting Dr. Phil, I was at ease. I talked freely and answered his questions honestly. There was no judgment, and I was able to share the things I worried about and the past hurts I was struggling to overcome. I left the office feeling better than I had in months. I had let go of emotions I had been holding onto unnecessarily and felt lighter, clearer, calmer.

Hoyt and I agreed that speaking to this professional had been a positive experience. We had new strategies to help us handle the stress and uncertainty of the coming month. Dr. Phil gave us the green light. We were sane and we were stable.

Next came the orientation at the fertility clinic. Hoyt and I had been through this session once before and knew what to expect but dreaded it just the same. We sat quietly, staring grimly toward the blank projector screen at the front of the room, waiting for the presentation to begin. Meanwhile, Rhonda sipped her coffee and chatted pleasantly with the woman beside her, unaware of the overwhelming information and scary statistics she would hear over the next hour.

The clinic gathered all the couples scheduled for IVF during the upcoming cycle into a conference room together. Each doctor from the clinic took a turn presenting information. They taught about the IVF process, the odds of certain diseases and conditions, the needles and the drugs possible side effects, and what to expect throughout each procedure. I sat on my hard, plastic seat and tried to rationalize the frightening statistics while I scribbled down directions for how to mix drugs correctly and time injections perfectly. The information began to swirl around faster than I could take it in or write it down. Soon, my head began to swim.

The mood in the room quickly turned from expectancy and hope to confusion, which soon gave way to dread as we each realized what the next few weeks would hold. A quick glance at Rhonda revealed that she too was taken unaware by the gravity of the presentation. We made it through the training videos and alarming statistics about birth defects and success rates.

We ended the afternoon with one last consultation with Dr. Lucky Strike. This short appointment was the last opportunity that Hoyt, Rhonda, or I could take to ask our questions or gain reassurance.

Once again, I needed confirmation that Rhonda was healthy and I was normal, that this would work, that we had a chance, and that this was our best option. Again, Dr. Lucky Strike assured me our chances were good and everything was normal. Now, if we could simply sign here and just swipe our credit card there, we could begin the treatments. We signed and swiped and soon were out the door with two pink bags filled with fertility drugs—one for Rhonda and one for me.

The four of us piled into the truck that brilliant spring day with anticipation of what was to come in the following weeks. Talk of baby names and injection schedules consumed our conversations as busy city streets faded into the long stretches of open prairie that would take us home.

Our rollercoaster car was racing up the track in alignment with the steps in our fertility treatments. I felt the force of momentum push back on me, like a heavy weight on my chest, as the enormity of our decisions settled on my mind. In a few short weeks, I would be pregnant—finally. Rhonda was strapped into the seat beside me as the wind whipped her hair around her face. I closed my eyes, praying that I had made the right decisions and that we had chosen the right track.

As the treatment process steadily moved along, whispers of fear were like cold breath on the back of my neck. My intuition was reminding me to be cautious, to guard my heart, to prepare for the unexpected. I quietly ignored the whispers and murmurs of doubt. Instead, I pasted on a smile, and held on tight, just as I had so many times before.

Chapter 23

After the orientation, I was relieved to have a break from tests, appointments, and trips to the city. I was prescribed pills to take and needles to inject each evening. The needles were not as intimidating this time as I had given myself countless injections during my previous IVF cycle. I had an idea of what to expect and I didn't feel the same intensity of emotions or demand on my body the way I had in the previous cycle. I relaxed a bit.

Soak in every moment, I thought to myself. I wanted to remember each small detail so that one day, I could share memories of this time—their beginning—with our child.

I supported Rhonda as she bore the burden of this part of the cycle. It was easy for me to slide back into the role of bossy big sister as I pestered Rhonda with questions. Did you drink enough water today? Are you resting enough? You aren't lifting any heavy boxes at work, right? Do you have enough spinach at home? Did you inject your needle on time?

Rhonda handled the treatments, trips to the city, and my near-constant pestering with grace. She didn't complain once, even when her follicles had grown so large it was painful for her to bend over or sit down.

The silver lining of this two-week span during treatments, was time with my sister. Rhonda would stay overnight when she had early morning appointments in the city because our house was halfway between where she lived and where the fertility clinic was located. We would cook healthy dinners like zucchini noodles and meat sauce or make big nutritious salads. Only the best would do for my sweet sister and the eggs that would one day become our beautiful blond babies.

In the evening, we would do a cardio workout in my living room, sweating like crazy, to Rhonda's latest exercise video. Other times, we would try meditation; it was usually short lived because my dog would think we were trying to play with him, so our sessions would often lead to us laying on the floor playing with Ben instead.

Nothing made Hoyt leave for the safety of the shop, his truck, or the tractor faster than us in workout gear, laughing in the living room, our ponytails bouncing. In these moments, we were not just big sister and little sister. For the first time, we enjoyed each other as friends, confidantes, and equals. Our bond was stronger than ever.

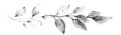

Have you had one of those mornings where you find yourself in your underwear, staring into the vast depths of your closet, complaining to your unconcerned husband who is still lounging in bed that you have nothing to wear?

Well, if you're like me, this scenario is all too common.

In my house, the usual sleepy suggestion from under the covers is that I should wear jeans and a shirt because that's what Hoyt was planning to wear. The fact that Hoyt can roll out of bed, jump in the shower, get dressed and be out the door in under fifteen minutes looking put together—whether he's going to the pasture or attending a wedding—did not help my mood on this particular morning. This morning was different. It was the morning of Rhonda's egg retrieval.

Daybreak had dawned, bright and clear on this special day. It was most certainly not just a jeans-and-a-shirt kind of day. I was up early because my nerves were tingling with excitement while my stomach flip-flopped nervously. I couldn't lay in bed for one moment longer. I was up and showered, the coffee was on, but I could not seem to pick an outfit to wear for the day.

It might seem trivial that I was worried about what to wear when we had the egg retrieval to contemplate, and you're right, it was. I couldn't wrap my head around whether a dress or capri pants would be more appropriate. I needed to find the perfect outfit to wear on this momentous day—the day the tiny little eggs that would soon become my babies were being retrieved from my sister's ovaries by a long needle in a dark and sterile procedure room. My mothering instincts were acting in full force as I threw one piece of clothing after the other onto the floor of my closet. You see, I knew what to wear if it was my son's first birthday or my sweet daughter's ballet recital, but what would a mom wear to an egg retrieval?

I finally settled on an appropriate outfit—a navy dress with a jean jacket and strappy sandals and I was ready to go. It was a beautiful spring morning, full sunshine in an endless blue sky, soft, cool breeze, and brilliant green grass. The energy of that gorgeous morning made me feel as though everything was right in my world. We left the house brimming with hope, anticipation, and excitement. We felt fully confident the procedure would go as planned, and this step of the process would soon be over.

Soon after the egg retrieval was completed and my sister was resting comfortably, our nurse, Evelyn, allowed Hoyt and me to go back to the recovery room to sit with Rhonda as she was waking up. I will never forget the walk down that hallway. I was a bundle of nerves, barely able to contain my curiosity and tangible need to know the results of the retrieval. Evelyn informed us the procedure had gone well. Dr. Lucky Strike had been able to retrieve ten viable eggs.

Ten viable eggs. Ten chances. Ten reasons to hope. Ten reasons to finally be able to breathe.

Those ten perfect little eggs would soon be mixed with Hoyt's donation and the wonder of fertilization would begin. The process was working. The sunshine streamed in through the windows in the recovery room as if proof that everything was right. We marvelled at the science and the divine wonder that is involved in creating life.

The next few days were nerve-wracking. We were home and trying to carry on as usual even though nothing was truly normal. Hoyt, Rhonda, and I were all on edge, tense, and waiting. We wondered and worried and hoped. Would the eggs fertilize? Was my body ready for implantation? Would this work? Would Hoyt and I finally become parents?

I was at work when my phone rang. It was the embryologist from the fertility clinic, calling to tell me how many of Rhonda's eggs were fertilized. I answered the phone with trepidation. It is easier in some ways not to know because I could still hope and expect. There is still a chance. The embryologist explained that only three out of ten of our eggs fertilized. They were watching the embryos to see whether they were developing as expected. I hung up the phone, devastated. Only three embryos. How could that possibly be?

Rhonda does yoga every morning. She is young and healthy, and she eats things like quinoa and raw almonds. Hoyt's tests all came back with perfect scores. We all took vitamins, refrained from alcohol, and had plenty of rest. Dr. Lucky Strike had given us his assurances that everything would be fine. How could only three eggs have fertilized? We had been expecting all ten, or close to ten, would have been viable so we would have embryos to freeze for our "multiple future pregnancies" as Dr. Lucky Strike had suggested. We had been planning to have more than one child and wanted some room for error; this was not part of our plan. I panicked immediately.

I called Hoyt and Rhonda to share the news as soon as I had finished speaking with the embryologist. Hoyt answered on the second ring.

"Hoyt, the embryologist just called. Only three eggs fertilized," I blurted into the phone. "Only three! But there were ten! How could this have happened?" I wailed.

Hoyt remained calm. He considered for a moment and then spoke slowly, "Well, we have three embryos. That's good news. Three embryos, three little babies are growing right now. I don't know why only three fertilized, honey, but it only takes one embryo to make a baby. We have three chances. Don't worry yet. Try to stay calm and we'll see what happens in the next few days," he reasoned.

We still had three chances. Don't give up; don't lose hope. I went home after work that night cautiously optimistic and entirely focused on preparing my body for those precious embryos. My rollercoaster had long since left the gate and we were gearing up for the ascent to the highest point of this heart-racing, stomach-dropping, twisting and turning ride that was my life.

Chapter 24

I have observed the beauty and diversity of motherhood throughout my life—from South Korea to Canada. Urban, rural, rich, poor—the beauty of motherhood and the language of that instinctive love is always the same. I marvel at the miracle that is motherhood in all its glory. I am in awe of the bond a mother has with her child. I soak in the stories of what it is like to experience pregnancy and to feel life beating beneath your heart. I ache to know what it is like to hear my child cry for the first time or to call me "Mommy." I imagine the feeling of a baby curled and sleeping, safe and sound, against my breast. I dream of the moment I can share with my husband and my family that I am pregnant.

For eleven days, I was blessed to experience motherhood and the power of loving my children. I was overcome by the fierce intensity of motherly protection for my unborn babies. I revelled in the feeling of my husband whispering, "I'm so proud of you," with his hand placed protectively on my stomach. I was a mother for eleven glorious days. Two of our embryos were perfect. Healthy. Thriving. I was carrying those perfect, healthy, thriving babies. I finally understood what it was like to hold life within my body. Pure, sweet, joy vibrated through my soul with the knowledge that I held our children in my womb. At last I was carrying the babies that my husband and I so desperately wanted and already loved. Sweet, liquid, pulsing relief ran through me and washed away the heartache, hurt, fear, and worry I had endured during the seven long years of my infertility.

Our excitement was palpable. We couldn't contain it. We planned; we talked; we dreamed; we expected. We firmly believed I was carrying twin boys. Hoyt and I laughed about what trouble two mischievous Colven boys would cause and bantered back and forth over who would have to go to the school to sort it out when we received those inevitable calls. We decided how we would arrange two cribs, not just one, in the spare bedroom reserved to soon become our nursery. I spent hours choosing paint colors and quilt patterns to decorate our babies' room. I imagined rocking two crying babies in the middle of the night and how I wouldn't mind losing sleep one bit.

We poured over baby names, exploring different combinations and scoffing at one another's choices until we finally settled on two names. Boys' names, of course, because Hoyt was convinced our babies were boys. Hoyt had big plans for all the things he would do with his sons. We studied the pictures of our embryos with amazement, trying to imagine how those clusters of cells would one day soon become our children. I planned the perfect way to announce our news to our families and what catchy phrase I could put on onesies as a reminder these babies were special. Our boys had a long journey to come into the world. I couldn't wait to put all our plans into action.

I understood it now. I understood what it meant to feel the unconditional love, the instant bond, the fierce protectiveness that comes with motherhood. Hoyt and I tenderly held onto our special secret—our babies were on their way. We felt connected to each other on a totally new level of intimacy. We both knew the sacrifices and science that it had taken for me to hold these two tiny miracles inside my body. With the realization that I was carrying our babies, the longing to become a mother that I had valiantly tried to quiet when childlessness was a looming reality came bubbling up to the surface and exploded out of my soul. It was transformational. In eleven days, my life changed forever.

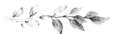

Dr. Lucky Strike had recommended bed rest after the embryo transfer was complete and I dutifully obeyed his orders. For the first two days, I relaxed in bed. I was sore and achy from the transfer procedure and my body felt heavy and swollen due to the fertility hormones coursing through my body. My day was scheduled around progesterone suppositories morning, noon, and night, prescribed to assist my body in holding onto this precious pregnancy. By day three, sore and achy turned into dull cramping in my lower abdomen. I was hypervigilant to any twinge I felt, unsure of what was "normal" and what was concerning. My senses were on high alert for the first sign of nausea which could be morning sickness, or a heightened sense of smell, or cravings for certain foods—any sign that I might be pregnant.

By day seven, my cramping was accompanied by an ominous, brown discharge which, over the course of the next two days, turned to the most unwelcome sight—spots of bright red blood. *No, no, no, no, no!* was all my terrified brain could shout. I anxiously searched my discharge papers for possible alternatives to the reality that I could be losing my babies. Relief came when I read that spotting, discharge, and even light bleeding could be considered "normal" after an embryo transfer. I rationalized that my spotting was really implantation bleeding and that my babies were safe. The cramps continued and my spotting turned to bleeding. Bright red blood on pure white fabric. Try as I might, I couldn't convince my brain or my heart that it was only an implantation bleed. Raw, hot, fury engulfed me. Fear of losing my babies consumed every waking thought and every uneasy dream at night. The next three days were possibly the longest of my life. I laid perfectly still in my bed, progesterone oozing out of me, willing the hormones to work and praying that my miracle babies could hold on. I bartered with God. I begged. I cried. I prayed some more. *Let my babies live.*

Then came day twelve.

Day twelve was the day we would know for certain whether our dreams had come true and I was pregnant. Dr. Lucky Strike had given me a requisition form for an hCG blood test which would determine if our transfer had been successful. Hoyt and I dressed silently, lost in our own thoughts, as we prepared for this important day. We drove to the city, cautious, hopeful, and anxious.

"Do you think I'm pregnant?" I gingerly asked Hoyt. I wasn't sure if I wanted to hear his answer.

"It says in the discharge papers that bleeding is normal. There's still hope, honey. Our twins are strong, the embryos were perfect, remember?" Hoyt urged me to stay positive. His innocent insistence that we cling to hope broke my heart. I knew that the bleeding that had started was not normal, even if I didn't want to admit it to myself, much less to my husband.

Hoyt pulled into a parking spot in front of the medical clinic and gave my hand a squeeze. I sat for a moment and tried to clear my head. I was so terrified to walk into the lab because I knew that the answer to my question of pregnancy was one blood test away. Not knowing a definitive answer allowed room for hope and rationalization to reign. This truly was our last chance and I was unprepared for a negative result. I squared my shoulders and walked inside. I had to know for sure if I was pregnant or not.

A quick blood test was followed by hours of agonizing waiting for the phone call that would give us the results of my hCG test.

Hoyt and I decided to stay in the city for the day while we waited. We tried and failed to keep our thoughts from racing. It was then, during the waiting that doubt and fear flooded our dreams. What if the test came back negative? What if it hadn't worked?

Hoyt put the truck in gear and steered out of the clinic's parking lot. We ran a few errands and wandered through a few shops, trying to pass the time. Eventually, we found a coffee shop and sat silently together—Hoyt sipping strong, hot coffee and me drinking herbal tea—each lost in our own thoughts. It was a long, quiet morning, each of us contemplating possible outcomes, waiting for the phone to ring.

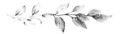

The call came in the middle of lunch. I saw the number for Dr. Lucky Strike's office pop up on my phone. It was loud in the restaurant, so I stepped outside to take the call. It was our nurse, Evelyn, from the fertility clinic. We exchanged the required pleasantries, and then she said the words that still haunt me today. I had fervently prayed for a positive answer to my motherhood prayers. But it would not be so. Evelyn's words initiated the chain reaction that forced my baby rollercoaster over the height of my joy and sent it careening down the track to utter destruction.

"I'm sorry. Your pregnancy test came back negative. You aren't pregnant, Janice. You can stop taking the progesterone suppositories. Dr. Lucky Strike will see you in two weeks. Call and make an appointment. Have a nice day."

That was it. Factual. Black and white. No more wondering. I was not pregnant. Nothing could've prepared me to hear Evelyn's words.

Time stopped. Darkness clouded my vision. An invisible fist squeezed my chest so that I couldn't fill my lungs with air. My muscles were slow and unresponsive. My hands shook. I slowly stumbled back inside to our table and sat down in a heap. Hoyt looked at me expectantly, waiting for the good news. I couldn't speak. My tongue refused to form the words *not pregnant*.

I reluctantly met Hoyt's expectant gaze, dreading the moment that he would know that I had lost our twins. I hung my head and shook it slowly. No. I sat for a minute, the world spinning around me as the reality that my babies were dead descended on my consciousness, heavy and dark. The noise of the lunchtime crowd, the clanging of dishes, and the pulsating music in the background shattered into my stunned thoughts. How could anyone be laughing or visiting or eating their lunch right now? My world had stopped in an instant with one phone call.

Hoyt set his sandwich down on his plate, motioned for the waitress, and directed her to bring boxes for our food and the bill as quickly as possible. Then, he reached across the table and squeezed my hand. "Are you ok, honey? Say something. Tell me what Evelyn said on the phone. Honey? Jan? You have to talk to me." Hoyt pressed.

My voice was caught, strangled in my throat. I couldn't respond. I sat in silence as Hoyt dealt with the bill and our uneaten lunch. "Come on, honey. Let's get out of here," he said as he took my limp hand in his strong one.

Once in the truck, the tears came and I was powerless to stop them. Tears turned into sobs as I recounted the phone call that had rendered us childless. I wept as my heart was breaking and pouring out of me. "Well, now we know," was all Hoyt said as he drove through the city streets, jaw clenching and unclenching. It scared me to watch Hoyt's stoic reaction, unsure of what lay beneath his steely resolve of emotional strength. I was so overwhelmed by my own emotions, I never asked Hoyt how he felt. To be honest, I was scared of his answer. As the enormity of our new reality settled onto my heart like a black cloud, my tears fell faster and harder.

Chapter 25

We didn't speak on our way home. I wept from the depths of my soul the entire forty-five-minute drive. At one point, I glanced over at Hoyt and discovered tears streaming down his face as well. I had never seen Hoyt cry prior to this. His tears brought an uneasy and fearfully nauseating feeling to my stomach. To know I was the reason that Hoyt's heart was breaking cut to my soul.

To this point, Hoyt had always been the strong one. He was realistic, rational, calm, and my rock. A problem solver by nature, he always seemed to have an answer or know how to handle each new and challenging situation as it arose throughout our baby rollercoaster ride. I had never seen him fall apart and the thought of him doing so terrified me. If Hoyt was not able to be strong, if he didn't have the answer to our childlessness, then the loss, grief and pain must really be horrible—far too much to bear.

It was the first time in seven years of infertility that I felt truly alone and helpless. I was terrified to my core. I dreaded the implications of childlessness. I crumbled with guilt knowing that I had singlehandedly taken away Hoyt's chance to become a father. I feared that my marriage would dissolve because of the hell of infertility and that I would be left completely alone. I shuddered at the thought of once again rebuilding my life—this time without any hope of motherhood in my future.

Waves and waves of utter devastation washed over me in the days after my negative pregnancy test. Hoyt was sullen and quiet. We barely spoke, and if we did, it certainly wasn't about our lost twins. The pain was too fresh and too raw.

As if to rub salt in my wounded heart, I started bleeding heavily as soon as I stopped taking the fertility drugs. I no longer needed the progesterone suppositories to prevent miscarriage—my womb was empty. My body was rebelling against the unwelcomed hormones I had injected and swallowed day after day. Pain ripped through my abdomen in a cruel reminder of what I had lost as menstrual cramps rid my empty uterus of its lining. Blood ran between my legs in a steady stream, dark red, and accusing—washing away any trace of my babies. Pain, heavy bleeding, and cramps lasted for ten days—each day a miserable token of my immeasurable loss.

The fertility drugs had left my already heightened emotions in a jumbled heap that I tried—and failed—to untangle. I hated myself. My body had forsaken me. God had not been merciful. My prayers had been left unanswered. I was bitter and incredibly furious. It wasn't fair. I believed I had failed as a woman, as a mother, and as a wife. I could not protect my babies and I could not give my husband what he longed for and expected from me.

It just wasn't fair.

Despair and hopelessness settled over me like a cold, wet blanket. I sank into myself and my sorrow—unwilling to be vulnerable or to share how I felt with anyone. No one could possibly understand how I felt—or so I believed. I rarely expressed to Hoyt the depth of my sadness—I didn't have to—he felt it, too. Rhonda was the only person with whom I shared my true emotions. I called her each morning on my commute. She stayed on the phone with me while I sobbed my way to work and tried as best she could to comfort my inconsolable heart. Rhonda held her own secret sorrow—our twins belonged to her as much as they had belonged to Hoyt and me. My sadness seemed endless.

I wanted to stay in bed and hide. I hated myself more each day. I struggled to accept that I wasn't pregnant and probably would not ever be pregnant. I was furious we had spent all that money, involved my sister, and poured our hearts into this vision of our future family, only to be left with nothing but heartache and bills. I felt like I was being punished, and at the same time, I needed to punish myself. I felt solely responsible for our loss.

My heart hurt in a way I had never known it could hurt. I had experienced grief before, the loss of my father and grandparents, but that was nothing compared to the anguish and grief I was experiencing now.

For weeks after receiving my negative pregnancy results, involuntary tears would stream down my face or a sob would catch in my throat. For months, my throat felt tight and my head hurt. I moved mindlessly through my days in a mental fog. It was as if I was watching myself from outside my body. I lost interest in everything in my life. I couldn't be fully present. It was just too painful.

Chapter 26

My marriage was in trouble. As rational adults, Hoyt and I both knew my infertility and the loss of our twin boys was not my fault. A negative outcome had been a possibility all along, even though we had refused to consider that possibility. I felt extreme guilt for losing our babies, for killing our babies, for not being enough for our babies, and in turn, not being enough for my husband. I worried that Hoyt blamed and resented me. Hoyt's family farm and the legacy of his ancestors was in jeopardy. Hoyt would not have a son or an heir to continue the tradition of ranch life or to keep the heritage of his family farm alive. I could do nothing to fix the situation or make it right.

We fought.

We tried to come up with solutions, some realistic, some unconventional, none on which we could both agree. We wondered if our loss had occurred because we would not be good parents, or if we were being punished for some horrible thing we had done in the past. We asked ourselves if we were physically incompatible because no matter how hard we tried, our bodies could not produce a child together despite drastic medical intervention. Our minds went to these dark places and the stories we concocted pushed us further and further apart.

Finally, I offered to grant Hoyt a divorce, an out, another chance to find love and create a family with a fertile wife who could provide him the family he wanted. He declined my desperate offer, but our marriage was still rocky.

I cried and Hoyt withdrew. I became increasingly distant and moody. Hoyt lashed out with angry bursts. We were each grieving our loss and each trying to process it in our own way. Hoyt and I had always worked through our problems together, sharing everything. But this we couldn't do together. Our journey through the stages of grief was a journey we each had to walk alone. I prayed Hoyt would be able to find the patience and love to wait for me while I found my way through my sorrow.

My grief felt boundless and isolating. Now that I had had a taste of what my life could have been like, the future I almost had, I wanted more. Nothing seemed to compare to this life—a life of children and parenthood—for which I yearned. It felt like a cruel joke, a tease, to let me glimpse, to grant me eleven magnificent days of motherhood and then steal it away in an instant. I felt like the Universe was punishing me, laughing at me.

No one understood how I felt and I did not know how to make them understand. I felt like I would never be enough, never be able to give enough to make up for losing our babies.

It was impossible to rationalize what had gone wrong in our treatments. We had followed Dr. Lucky Strike's directions and our drug protocols religiously. We had done everything right. We had been incredibly sure, hopeful, and happy—then in a matter of seconds, everything we had dreamed of was crushed, gone forever.

I didn't know how to rebuild from here, how to go on, or how to be okay again. What was scarier to me was that I wasn't sure I even cared if I rebuilt or if I ever moved on to accept my childless life. I was depleted. I had nothing left to give and nothing for which to live. My baby rollercoaster car had jumped the track and crashed to smithereens, only a few feet from the exit gate. My unwelcomed ride left my weary spirit broken and alone, down in the depths of despair.

Chapter 27

Eight days after our heartbreak, Hoyt's brother and his wife welcomed a beautiful, perfect, precious baby girl into the world. My father-in-law was overjoyed at the birth of his new granddaughter.

The constant chatter was maddening. "Hey, Jan, how long are babies normally when they are born? Isn't this the most beautiful baby? Look at this picture, isn't she adorable? She has the proudest papa I've ever seen! When are you going to see her? I bet you can't wait to hold that baby girl!"

My answers consisted of polite mumblings. "Mmmhmmm. Gee, I don't know." I would nod with my face turned so I could brush away my tears. I wanted to scream "ENOUGH!" and beg him to stop gushing over the baby in my presence because my broken heart couldn't feel joy and it terrified me.

You see, up until this point, we had not told any of our family about our egg donation, our embryo transfer, or our negative pregnancy result. Doug's innocent and excited questions broke the frayed threads holding me together and I finally had to tell him about our lost babies and why I could not answer his excited questions or participate in his ongoing baby chatter.

To be clear, I love our niece, and I am relieved my sister-in-law can experience the joy that comes with being a mother. Infertility is hell and I wouldn't wish it for any woman. I am grateful for this beautiful baby girl we were blessed to welcome into our family, but the sting in my heart was a constant reminder of what had been taken away from me and what I would never experience.

In some ways, I also thought I didn't deserve to love any baby because I could not love my own. I questioned why some women were so blessed with motherhood and I was not.

The first time I saw our niece, my heart skipped a beat. She was so tiny and so perfect. Hoyt and I studied her little pink face and saw features that mirrored both her parents. When I witnessed the wonder my brother and sister-in-law shared over their daughter, I was reminded once again of what I had lost. When I saw the longing in my husband's eyes as he held his niece for the first time, I was reminded yet again of what I had taken from him. I could not hold my niece or even touch her because the pain of my sorrow was too present, too palpable. It took over every sense of my body. I could not trust myself to hold the baby without tears streaming down my face. I didn't want to take away even one moment of pure joy from the rest of my family with my sadness.

A few weeks later, our family was blessed by the birth of another beautiful, perfect, healthy baby girl—Auraelia Quinn—a fourth child for my brother and his wife. Once again, the raw sting of my unspoken secret sorrow kept me from being present in the moment and sharing in the euphoria of the new baby. Instead, I felt anger, fear, bitterness, and to be honest, jealousy—as I compared my childless life and perceived lack with the abundance of our siblings' lives. I was often caught off guard by the strength of these emotions. I allowed my anger to sweep me away as I wallowed in self-pity.

The only place I felt I could breathe was at work. At school, I didn't have to think through my emotions. My teaching was black and white. Data was collected and decisions were made. I understood exactly what was expected of me. I could do my job and do it well without involving my heart. It was a relief. An escape.

My office was my sanctuary. I have special items that students have given me through the years and meaningful mementos I have collected along the way that make me feel secure, safe, and relaxed. I would go in early and stay late. There was nothing in my office at school that reminded me of my failure as a woman or of my sorrow. I could talk to my colleagues at work about regular things, work things, trivial things. I could avoid the tough conversations that were always waiting for me at home.

My chest hurt, my throat was tight, and I had a constant headache. I would cry on my hour-long commute to and from work each day. I would cry in the shower; I would cry in bed when Hoyt thought I was sleeping. There was so much hurt I couldn't keep it inside of me; it leaked out in my tears. I felt like I would never smile again. I went through my regular daily routine, but there, bubbling just below the surface, was always the terrifying monster of grief, regret, and always—endless sorrow.

I needed help—a professional to guide me through my emotions and help me to heal. Instead, I stubbornly continued to wallow in my grief and continued to blame myself. I searched for comfort in old familiar habits and found myself using food to buffer my emotions. It didn't seem to matter how much I ate, the hole in my heart was never filled, never satisfied.

The layers of emotion resulting from infertility are as numerous as they are complex. The aftermath of infertility is difficult to navigate alone—as I experienced first-hand. Talking to a counsellor was one of the first and necessary steps I needed to take to begin working through my experience and find healing.

Six months after losing our embryos it was obvious that I was struggling. The darkness of my grief and the dangerous place that my spirit had settled, scared me. Depression consumed me. There seemed to be no conceivable way out of my grief. I wallowed in self-pity and soon became despondent. I lost interest in things had previously brought me joy. I rarely had the energy to even fake a smile. My relationships suffered as I shut the people who mattered most to me completely out of my life. My depression went on for months and worsened with each passing day.

When my mental state hovered precariously on the verge of suicidal, Hoyt urged me to make an appointment with the psychologist we had met earlier on our fertility journey. It was obvious that I could not pull myself out of my grief alone—so I made the call.

It very likely saved my life.

My counsellor helped me to work through each stage of my grief. While my experience with infertility was unique, my experience with grief was not uncommon. At each session, I talked through how I felt and the things that worried me the most. I learned strategies that helped me cope. My counselling remained ongoing after we ultimately walked away from fertility treatments and adoption—childless. Seeking support for my mental health was a crucial step in my healing.

After digging deeper into my grief to try to understand it, I learned I was experiencing something called "disenfranchised grief." According to Kenneth Doka, this is the grief a person experiences when they suffer a loss that is not or cannot be openly acknowledged, socially sanctioned or publicly mourned. I felt like no one understood or had empathy for my loss—not my family, and certainly not my community. I wasn't supposed to grieve because I didn't have a physical baby in my arms to mourn. There was no funeral—no one even knew we were going through fertility treatments at that time. These were just "fantasy babies" as someone once insensitively referred to my children. If that was true, then why couldn't I move on and just let it go?

Infertility is a multifaceted diagnosis. Unless you experience it yourself, you can't fully comprehend or anticipate its implications. I was not only grieving for my lost children but for my lost future. I was grieving for my husband's loss. I was grieving for every Christmas morning we would wake up to a quiet house that Santa had not visited. I was grieving for our vacant nursery and for the beautiful quilt that would never know the warmth of a sleeping baby. I was mourning our lonely supper table. I was grieving for the early morning snuggles, the bedtime stories, the tractor rides, and the school lunches I would never prepare. I was grieving my life and the future I thought was mine from the time that I was a child. I was lamenting the fact that I wouldn't be giving my mom grandchildren—a gift that she claims is her greatest joy in life. I mourned that I would never know motherhood.

Whenever someone in my family or community experiences a loss, I bring food, usually my famous lasagna. I call to check in on them, I attend the funeral, or I send a card and flowers. When I was at my lowest point—suffocating in grief—no one brought me a lasagna, sent me a card, or came to visit—because no one knew about my loss. The people who did know about my loss didn't know how to comfort me. There were no family and friends surrounding me, supporting me, helping me through the pain. There was no funeral to say goodbye. I felt alone in my grief with no idea how to move forward.

I needed closure, but I didn't know how to let go of my anger and my sadness so that I could move forward. After eight months of grieving, I would finally begin to find the closure I needed—and it came in the most unwelcome of ways.

Chapter 28

"Hysterectomy" is an emotionally charged word. It symbolizes a shift—a new definition of yourself as a woman. In my case, it was an unwelcomed shift—one against which I actively rebelled. Redefining myself as a childless woman had been difficult. Expanding that definition to include hysterectomy was overwhelming. More of my womanhood was being taken from me—against my will—and I didn't know if I could bear to lose anything else.

Eight months had passed since that fateful phone call in July informing me of my negative pregnancy test. In that time, I had worked hard to heal emotionally, but physically, I was in debilitating pain. I bled heavily for ten or more days at a time and rarely had relief from my pain—period or not. I decided to call and make an appointment to see Dr. Straight Shooter.

Dr. Straight Shooter raised the subject of a hysterectomy with me in her usual matter-of-fact style. She reasoned that there was just too much damage to my uterus to save it. It would never function normally nor would I ever carry a child. Endometriosis had fused my pelvic organs, jeopardizing their functioning, and sentencing me to a life of pain. The scarring was so severe that there was a good chance I would require a bowel dissection and a colostomy bag in addition to a hysterectomy. Dr. Straight Shooter's words jolted me to attention. "Hysterectomy" and "colostomy bag" were not terms I had been expecting to hear. She scheduled me for a hysterectomy in six short weeks and handed me a packet of information covering the basics of life with a colostomy.

Numbly, I signed the surgery consent documents as I listened to Dr. Straight Shooter describe the surgery and the risks. As she began to detail the necessary steps for the bowel dissection, creation of the stoma, and then the process for attaching a wafer and pouch, my consciousness shifted to somewhere outside of my body. I hovered in the air, watching the scene unfold below. I saw the scared, shell of a woman I had become and my spirit ached for her. My wish for the kind, loving, generous soul in the vision below was for her to walk boldly into her childless life—happy and whole, to love herself again, and to find her purpose beyond her infertility.

Dr. Straight Shooter ended our appointment that day with a firm handshake and these words, "I know it's difficult, Janice. It's the right decision for you medically and emotionally. Your quality of life will improve. You've lived in pain long enough. I'll see you in six weeks."

I left the doctor's office in a daze—shocked that Dr. Straight Shooter had rendered a hysterectomy as the necessary next step in my infertility journey. I didn't feel ready. I was so young for a hysterectomy—only thirty-three years old—and it was such a drastic and final step.

As my surgery date crept closer and the gravity of my situation set in, I became more and more distraught. The possibility of a colostomy bag was terrifying. I felt like I had lost so much already and now I might lose my dignity as well. I worried Hoyt would find me repulsive, or worse, that I would *be* repulsive. I feared I would wake up no longer a woman, in menopause, with a colostomy bag, chin whiskers, and a dry vagina.

It was a reality to which I did not want to wake.

How had my life fallen so far off the path I had planned for myself? Life wasn't supposed to be like this! My impending surgery stirred up all the fear, anger, and bitterness I had spent many months trying to suppress. No matter how hard I tried to contain my emotions and pretend I was doing fine, my body kept score, and it didn't forget. My tears flowed freely once again, except this time, they were tears wishing I wouldn't wake up to my new reality. I refused to redefine my life again post-hysterectomy. I was tired. Tired of hurting. Tired of fighting. Tired of feeling cheated and bitter.

I was done.

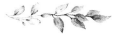

My surgery was again scheduled for the middle of calving season so Hoyt had to stay on the ranch. My sweet sister said yes, of course, she would come and stay with me while I was in the hospital. Rhonda and I left home early on that cold March morning to arrive at the hospital on time.

Waiting for my surgery was excruciating. Anxiety ruled my mind and the long hours of waiting forced me to imagine the worst. My unease grew with each moment as we raced down lonely stretches of icy, black highway to the city that held my fate.

There was no witty banter in my pre-op room. This time, I laid dejectedly in my hospital bed—angry tears racing hot tracks down my cheeks. I dreaded the moment I would walk into Dr. Straight Shooter's operating room for one final surgery—the one that would take my final essence of womanhood.

Waking up from surgery this time was like coming out of an inky black dream. I couldn't seem to open my heavy eyelids. When I did, it was to a world that was too bright and loud. My head ached, and there was a thick, sick, feeling in my stomach. I wished I could go back to sleep.

From the depths of my dream, I heard an echoing voice saying, "Janice, Janice, wake up, breathe. Come on, wake up, your surgery is finished. You're in the recovery room now."

I didn't recognize the voice and I refused to open my eyes. I heard my name again and realized I had no choice; I had to wake up—the nurse would continue to call my name until I did. My eyes slowly squinted open to a room bustling with nurses, bright lights, and beeping machines. I slowly awoke to the cold, harsh reality of post-hysterectomy life. It was the moment I would find out if my fears of a colostomy bag had come true or if I had been spared.

Instantly, I was awake and desperate for the answer.

In a shaky voice, I asked my nurse, "Do I have a colostomy bag?"

"Let's take a look," came her reply. The nurse cautiously lifted a corner of my sheet to reveal my body underneath. It only took a second for her to determine that there was no bag. "No colostomy bag," she answered cheerfully. "Just a hysterectomy for you today."

I was floating in the space between half conscious, half dreaming, and I couldn't be sure I had heard correctly. Her answer seemed too hasty. Had I heard wrong? Had she looked carefully? Although, I'm not sure how you could miss a colostomy bag.

"Check again. Check the other side," I demanded.

She laughed and obliged. "There is no bag!" she assured me. I settled back against my stark, white, hospital pillow, and let the news sink in.

Her words were sweet music to my ears. I couldn't believe it was true. The weeks of worry, expecting the worst, the endless nights spent sleepless and sobbing in anticipation of this surgery had all been for naught.

I had been so focused on the perceived adverse outcome that I hadn't allowed myself to hope. I had forgotten that yes, a colostomy bag was a real possibility, but it was not the only possibility. There was, of course, the chance that my surgery would be routine, I would recover quickly, and would feel infinitely better than I had before. So why had my brain—as well as my heart—conspired to prepare me for the worst?

Seven years of disappointment had conditioned me to expect the worst, to plan for it, and to not even dare hope or consider the positive. It felt like whenever my doctor would claim that 99% of cases were successful, I would be the 1% for whom the procedure would fail—every time.

Hoping was a dangerous game that I had lost playing time and again. I had braced myself for the worst-case scenario—the kind of dismal outlook that had me purchase plain, unsweetened applesauce and pack my freezer full of the bland, pureed goop in preparation for life with a colostomy bag. The stories I told myself were dark, miserable, and far from factual. I wish, instead, I had been gentler with my soul and had reined in my wild imagination.

In those moments when everything seems out of control and scary and you don't want to carry on—breathe. There will be moments, hours, and days that will feel cruel and unending. Don't give up. Be gentle with yourself. Be aware of the story you're telling yourself. If the narrative running through your head on a continuous loop is hurting your heart, like mine was, stop! You are in control of your story, so love yourself. Even during the hormone craziness, heartbreak, disappointment, and sorrow of infertility, love yourself.

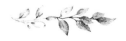

After two days in the hospital, I was able to go home—in one piece, fully functioning, and never more relieved. Darlene had come stay with us for a few days so she was with Hoyt when I arrived.

I burst in the door and took a deep breath. I was home. I was safe. I was going to be okay. I had left this house broken, scared, depressed, and in constant pain. I returned healthier, energized, vibrant, and confident. Something happened in that hospital room after my surgery. A shift in my mindset and a change in my heart occurred. The thought of living a pain-free life filled me with hope. My post-surgery pain was nothing when compared with the daily pain I had suffered for thirteen long years. It was invigorating. Positive energy was coursing through my soul, full of possibility for the future.

I took off my boots and coat and hurried to the bathroom in our bedroom. I opened cupboard doors and slammed drawers open and shut.

"What's going on?" I heard Darlene's bewildered voice coming from the kitchen.

I emerged from our bedroom with a red wicker basket. This basket had the distinct honour of holding my pads and tampons for the seven years of my marriage. For eighty-four months, this basket had witnessed my tears as I reached into its depths. This basket represented my disappointment with each negative pregnancy test and the searing pain caused by my endometriosis each cycle.

On this momentous day, I filled that horrible crimson-colored basket with every tampon and pad, leftover fertility drug, prenatal vitamin, ovulation predictor, pregnancy test, and needle. I was determined and unstoppable as I tore up the colostomy information packet into tiny pieces. Rhonda and Darlene watched in silence as I rooted through the junk drawer for a lighter, grabbed my coat and boots, and headed outside into the cold and gloomy March afternoon. It wasn't the sort of thing a recent surgery patient was expected to do.

My mission was simple. I needed the reminders of my infertility out of my life and out of my sight—immediately. I met Hoyt coming down the lane. He followed me to our fire pit with suspicion written all over his face. Usually, the fire pit is reserved for backyard barbeques and late summer wiener roasts.

Today, it was to be the scene of a cleansing.

Determined, I set my basket of infertility and broken dreams into the fire pit and sprinkled the tiny bits of colostomy information over the top. With a hiss of the lighter, the shreds of paper instantly caught and burst into a glowing flame. That one small flame grew larger and licked at the edges of the wicker basket until it erupted into flames and suddenly, there was a roaring fire, blazing before me.

Each crackle and pop empowered me. Something beautiful was happening to my soul. I was letting go. Finally, the weight I had carried in my heart for seven long years was lifting; I could feel it leave my body. Infertility was no longer my reality, my failure, my grief. I could move on. I could live my life as a confident and vibrant woman full of grace and strength. At that moment, I knew I would be okay, that we would be okay.

Hoyt and I watched our fire burn until it slowly fizzled out. I turned to him, tears streaming down my cheeks. My sweet husband kissed my tears away, took my hand, and led me back to our house. Hoyt is my husband, my family, and my love. It became so clear to me in that moment that my purpose was to love him and to enjoy this life that we have been given, with or without children.

We walked back to the house, hand in hand, and for the first time in seven years, I felt truly at peace. That cleansing fire was the closure for which my soul had been longing. It was the end of that part of my life—my ride on my baby rollercoaster was over. I could finally put my infertility to rest and move on—childless. I entered our house surrounded by the love of my husband and my family. I was empowered and determined to find my purpose beyond motherhood and to live a meaningful life.

Chapter 29

I love dogs. They are loyal and protective—and happy to see you when you come home.

My first dog was a rescue animal that my dad picked out for me on my fourth birthday. He was a big black dog with long hair. He must have been a pampered house dog at some point because he seemed to dislike farm life. He preferred to sleep in a cozy corner of our living room, curled up in the sunshine, than to run around outside. His long, black hair was hot and he would pant as he tried to find a shady spot to lay during the heat of a summer day. In the winter, he avoided going outside altogether.

It was love at first sight for me. I named him Finny after the only other dog I knew—Mr. Dress-Up's puppet, Finnegan. Finny would be the first of many dogs that would find their way into my life at the exact time that I needed them.

After finishing my Bachelor of Education degree, I boldly accepted a contract to teach English abroad for a year—much to my parents' astonishment. This quiet, play-it-safe, farm girl was going to take on the world.

I met Nancy while I was teaching in a city on the southern tip of the Korean peninsula. One day, Nancy was walking down the street when something caught her eye. She looked again and what she saw made her stop. A little dog was darting this way and that to dodge vehicles on the busy Korean street. Nancy coaxed him to safety and picked him up. Then she did the only thing she could; she brought him home.

Nancy was not a dog person. She asked if I would take care of the animal until she could decide what to do with him. I enthusiastically agreed. I bathed him and fed him. This messy, yappy little dog found his way into my heart instantly. He was grateful to be warm, clean, fed, and safe, and I was thankful for his snuggles, wet dog kisses, and companionship. I named him Ben and he went everywhere with me, including home to Canada when I finished my year of teaching in South Korea.

The next dog in my life would be *our* dog not just *my* dog. Hoyt and I brought Riley, our brown and white Australian Shepherd, home the first December we were together. He had one blue eye and one brown eye and a personality as big as the great outdoors. We loved him instantly. Riley was smart and sweet. He brought humor and light to our household and was the perfect dog for us.

A few years later, my mother-in-law, Darlene, called to tell us her next-door-neighbor was moving and a new home was needed for her dog, Trigger. A beautiful fox-red, Labrador, Trigger was a trained hunting dog, great with kids, and he needed a new home, fast. Hoyt was shaking his head while I was on the phone; he already knew what was coming.

As soon as I hung up, he said, "No, we were not getting another dog. Riley and Ben are enough."

I, on the other hand, felt quite sure we had room in our house and our hearts for one more dog. Hoyt relented after listening to me plead my case. One week later, we were a three-dog family. I felt justified that if I wasn't able to fill my house with children that I could logically fill it with dogs instead.

Trigger came home to us but he never quite fit in with our family. He was frisky and rambunctious. He craved attention and would often jump into your lap, all slobbery and unwelcome 100 pounds of him. Other times, when the door was opened, he would run you over trying to get out of the house—and he would keep running and not come back. We spent hours searching the countryside for Trigger and bringing him back home.

On one of his trips away, Trigger followed his nose to our little town, about four miles from home. He worked as a greeter outside the local grocery store for the afternoon until one of the cashiers called to let us know that Trigger was safe and could we please come and collect him.

Trigger was terrified of thunderstorms, of which we had many that summer. He would howl, cry, and scratch at the door hours before a storm, even when the sky was still blue and the sun was shining. He would bark and run in circles, crying frantically once the storm hit. He was inconsolable and his behavior wore on our nerves. We did not know what to do with him, how to comfort him. Nothing seemed to work.

Trigger caused us stress and cost us a fortune. He chewed everything including a brand new dog bed, stuffing and all. The only thing left was the trim from the edges. Hoyt's *I told you so,* expression appeared on his face every time Trigger chewed something else or ran away for the umpteenth time.

My husband was right to be annoyed. He never wanted another dog, but I forced the issue. I insisted, pestered, bugged, and whined until I had my way. It ended badly, for the dog and for us. Trigger is no longer a member of our family and I learned a valuable lesson. When something doesn't feel right, you should probably not force it. Dog adoption did not feel right. I had forced and coerced Hoyt to adopt Trigger.

Adopting a child at this point in our journey felt forced and coerced too. It felt as though our society was expecting that we should adopt, as though it was our duty as a childless couple. But for us, it just did not feel right.

During the years of our fertility treatments, conversations about our future changed from a resounding *when* we have children to a cautious *if* we have children. Most of these conversations were whispered in the dark, under the covers, because it was too scary to say them out loud in the bright daylight.

When it became apparent we were not on the societally-approved schedule to start our family, the advice began. It didn't seem to matter if I was at the dentist chatting with the hygienist or at a family event speaking to a relative, everyone had an opinion on our childlessness and what our options might be. One seemingly easy solution kept coming up in conversations with family and friends alike. *Why don't you just adopt?*

Just. Adopt.

Those two words should never be said together. The decision to adopt is life-changing and not one to make lightly. Nor can you *just adopt*. Adoption is not the quick and easy way to obtain a child that most of these well-meaning commenters think. There are many factors to consider and barriers to overcome. However, for a woman experiencing infertility, there is societal pressure, real or imagined, to adopt.

When this advice came up in conversation, I would mumble something about yes, it was an option, and yes, we would consider it. Then I would change the topic of conversation or leave the room as soon as possible, knowing that adoption was not right for us, at least not at that moment in time.

A colleague at my school was employed as a social worker before joining our school team. I have spoken to her about adoption many times. Hearing her talk of this precious experience is inspiring. Adoption is a beautiful thing, a noble thing. Giving a child a wonderful life, a life they would not otherwise have, feeling the joy their presence would bring to yours, is nothing short of a miracle. I deeply respect couples who adopt.

One of my fears was, if we did adopt, what if the child never felt like mine? What if we might not bond? Then what would I do? My friend reassured me that in all her years and the many adoptions she had facilitated, every baby she had placed in waiting arms was met with love and an instant bond. No one ever, even one time, said, "No, this is not my baby; I want a different one."

I could not shake the feeling that adoption was not right for us. After planning and expecting that one day I would carry a child below my heart, give birth to, and raise that perfect sweet baby, adoption seemed to pale in comparison. At least it did for me.

I longed to look at a child, our child, and see my husband's green eyes staring back at me. I ached to watch my child grow up, to see their personality unfolding, to understand their quirks, and to know they were just like me or just like Hoyt. I wanted desperately to give Hoyt a child that had Colven genes. I wanted to know my child's family medical history. Then I would know what to watch for, expect, and avoid with our child. How would I know how to protect a stranger's child? I had so many fears and still clung to the dream of having a child of my own.

Our situation was complicated by more than just wanting a child. Hoyt's farm had been in the family for over 100 years. Generations of Colvens had toiled and sacrificed to keep the farm running smoothly and ensure the land stayed in the family name. Hoyt had certainly sacrificed and worked tirelessly to keep his prairie roots and the Colven legacy—his legacy—alive.

The reality that he would not have an heir to pass this legacy on to was upsetting. Hoyt's sense of responsibility to all the strong pioneering men who had gone before him was overwhelming.

I felt guilty for standing in the way of a century-old tradition and family legacy. Adopting was not that simple for us. Yes, it would give us a chance to be parents, but an adopted child would not have Colven blood running through their veins.

Hoyt was adamant. Adoption did not feel right for him. I would not insist, pester, or plead my case for adoption. I had learned my lesson with the dog. If it did not feel right for both of us, we would not do it. A baby is forever; you cannot simply send it back if it doesn't fit in. It had to be right for both of us.

After engaging in an adoption conversation with someone, I would often feel guilty and angry. It seemed that because I was infertile, it was my responsibility to adopt and care for those children the rest of the world had overlooked. I felt guilty that there were children hurting and alone that we could have helped if we chose to adopt. I worried that the world was judging us for our decision.

I felt angry that I had been faced with the choice of whether or not to adopt. I was angry that I had been cheated out of motherhood. I was furious that family, friends, and strangers alike all seemed to think they should have an opinion about my life.

I wanted to ask, "Why did you decide to have a biological child? Why didn't you just adopt instead of having a baby of your own? The world is full of children without parents. You should have adopted too because it is everyone's responsibility to care for these children."

Of course, I never said this to anyone who was insisting adoption was the answer for me as it would have been both rude and insensitive. I said nothing and carried on quietly, adding this comment to the secret sorrow of my infertility.

Although we felt that adoption probably was not a choice we would make, Hoyt and I often considered our options and the possibility of adoption. We called the adoption center in our province, read all the information we could find, and went for an initial question and answer meeting with an adoption worker. We came home with a guidebook and a questionnaire to work through together. The guidebook outlined the adoption process in our province while the questionnaire guided us through conversations about each of our beliefs and concerns about adopting a child. Adoption seems like the easy answer for an infertile couple, but it is not easy at all. It is a complicated and intricate process.

We learned that we had three basic options if we chose adoption: a private adoption, a domestic adoption, or an international adoption. As we delved into the details of each type of adoption, the possibility seemed further and further out of our reach.

A private adoption meant we knew someone who had a child and wanted to place that child with us for adoption. This type of adoption was an arrangement of "chance" and would be done independently, outside of the adoption agency in our province. It was not an option that we could plan for in advance. We would be responsible for all the costly legal fees and would have to go through the lengthy adoption process—a process which could take years. The child's biological parents could change their minds for up to three weeks after all the necessary documents had been signed and consent to the adoption had been given. It sounded reasonable except we didn't know anyone who had a child and was willing to place it for adoption. These unknown factors fell like roadblocks on our path of becoming parents.

We moved on to investigate domestic adoption. Domestic adoption involves adopting a child who is in the care of the province. This type of adoption is paid largely in part by the province, which made it a more attractive option than private or international adoption. Children who are eligible for adoption through the province are usually older children who've often experienced trauma, a difficult start to their young lives, or have some special need. To adopt an infant, which is what we hoped, we would potentially be on the waiting list for up to seven long years.

I felt like we could love any child and could give that child a stable home and lots of love despite any diagnosis or history the child might bring. Hoyt was more realistic. He was worried about the challenges and struggles we would face raising a child not biologically ours and potentially with special needs or serious medical concerns. He was also concerned that if we were on the waiting list for seven years, we would be over forty years old before we even had the possibility of adopting, which wasn't something Hoyt was willing to do. We moved on to learn about international adoption.

International adoption seemed like it might be our best choice because adoptive parents had more control over the process. However, as we learned more, we discovered so many stumbling blocks that we quickly lost our enthusiasm. For example, to adopt a child from South Korea, you are required to be within a specific body mass index range. Some countries have age restrictions or financial expectations for adoptive parents. We discovered that international adoptions could cost upwards of $70,000, and there is still no guarantee we would be adopting the healthy infant for which we longed. In addition to the thousands of dollars we had already spent on fertility treatments, that astronomical cost seemed an insurmountable obstacle to our journey towards parenthood.

We started working through the questionnaires and conversation points outlined in our adoption guidebook. It became obvious that Hoyt and I were at different points in our healing and our commitment to adoption. Whenever we tried to envision our life with an adopted child, images of our own blond-haired, green-eyed baby boys came sharply into focus. That dream of our own children paired with the invasive look into the most intimate details of our lives and finances left us feeling vulnerable and exposed. These were feelings we had after only one initial intake meeting and an afternoon spent working through the adoption guidebook.

Hoyt and I continued having long, heart-to-heart talks about adoption and our childless reality. We half-heartedly continued to research adoption and to connect with other couples who had adopted.

Then, one day, we just stopped.

We were tired of trying so hard but always running into a wall. We believed that creating our family shouldn't be so difficult. We were tired of fighting, tired of having the same conversation repeatedly without finding solutions, tired of spending money we didn't have to pursue a dream that always seemed to be just out of our reach. We both realized it was time to stop chasing after the life we thought we were supposed to live and to love the life we had.

Throughout our time aboard our baby rollercoaster, the reality of my infertility was unforgiving. Even though we tried so hard, exhausting every unconventional avenue, our dream of parenthood remained unfulfilled. Slowly, the realization dawned that it might be time to change our dream. It might be time to surrender our expectations and what we thought we wanted so badly. We started listening to the whispers of our intuition and understood that "different" doesn't necessarily mean "bad." The Universe has a plan in store for us, just waiting to be revealed in perfect timing.

Chapter 30

Our culture assumes that during our childbearing years, all women are mothers and as we age, that all women are grandmothers. Expectations for what life looks like for a woman at each stage are woven into society's perception of our identity as women. We can all bring to mind images of a young mother holding her newborn baby or of a warm and matronly grandmother, arms open wide to welcome her throng of adoring grandchildren.

Phrases exulting women as mothers and grandmothers abound—*a mother's love, a face only a mother could love, forever and always, my baby you'll be, when you look in a mother's eyes, you see the purest love you can find on earth, giving birth is the most powerful act a woman can preform,* or *nothing beats being a grandma, happiness is being a grandma, being a grandma is as close as we get to perfection, grandchildren are the jewels of our golden years* and on and on it goes.

Society's perception of women as mothers is maintained by media, imagery, and by women ourselves. We see commercials selling diapers, coffee, even arthritis medication, portraying women as mothers and grandmothers. Songs play on the radio celebrating the joys of parenthood. Conversations at work and at leisure center on children and eventually, grandchildren—the cutest thing the child did, the extravagant birthday party, the excitement of winning the game. These proud moments shape our identities. Women compare sleepless nights, birth stories, hockey and dance schedules, the "terrible twos," and shopping for an endless list of September school supplies all as badges of honour and a necessary part of being a woman.

I am not a mother or a grandmother and my proud moments look differently. I often find it hard to relate to the experiences of women my same age. My accomplishments seem to hang on the periphery of the children-centered topics that dominate our conversations.

I have been asked on countless occasions how many children I have or if I have children. These questions are usually made unconsciously on behalf of someone who is clueless to the sorrow of infertility. They have no idea the emotion triggered by their simple questions. When I respond that I don't have children, the line of questioning and advice usually continues, "When are you planning on having children? You shouldn't wait too long to start your family."

It is simply assumed that because of my age, I am a mother. It's incorrect to assume that all women are mothers or grandmothers—we're not.

Throughout my infertility, Hoyt and I have both received insensitive comments, endless advice, and mindless remarks made by well-meaning people. *Just relax, and it will happen. Be patient. You can't rush these things. Have you tried going on vacation? Enjoy your freedom while it lasts. Maybe if you got more sleep you'd conceive. Have you tried raising your legs after sex? I have a great detox you should try. It must be those toxins that are causing your infertility. Grapefruit and herbal tea cured my infertility. My cousin has endometriosis and she has three children, you just have to keep trying. Have you thought about adoption?*

I've been offered these sage bits of wisdom—none of them are helpful. It wouldn't matter how many grapefruits I ate while relaxing on vacation with my legs in the air, enjoying my freedom and detoxing my toxins. At the end of that vacation, I'd return home to find that my endometriosis was still there. My womb—and my arms—eternally empty.

With every fiber of my soul, I wish I could take this advice, just relax, and end my infertility once and for all. The reality is—there's no escape. I can't "just relax" or "try harder" or wish my way to motherhood. This "advice" only caused me guilt, shame, and more anxiety—not comfort. I continued to carry my infertility with me wherever I went, secretly, hiding it from the world.

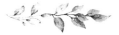

One summer day following my failed IVF cycle, I took a road trip with a friend. We stopped for a nice dinner at one of my favorite restaurants. The conversation was light and comfortable but eventually turned more meaningful and my infertility was the inevitable topic.

Sometimes, I would be angry and feel like no one cared if no one asked how I was doing or sympathized with me. At other times, I would be upset when someone did ask how I was doing because I felt like my infertility was too private, too painful and I was not strong enough to talk about my experience in more than a shaky whisper. On this evening, however, I felt safe and connected and so I shared my experience.

The restaurant was dimly lit with the gentle glow of flickering candlelight. There were white linens on the table and wine in our glasses. The bustle of the busy restaurant was a pleasant hum in the background of our conversation. The wine had dulled my senses a bit. I was relaxed and settled in to bare my soul. I shared my emotions, my fears for the future, and my frustrations with the unfair and unexpected turn my life had taken. I shared because I felt comfortable and loved and I wanted to be understood. For even a moment, I wanted someone besides my husband and sister to understand my secret sorrow. The conversation went like this:

"I am fearful we will never have a child. I am not sure my marriage could survive that. We have been through so much already. What if I am not strong enough to try another round of IVF?" I questioned.

The response came. "I'm sorry that you are going through this."

"Thanks, me too. I wish my life were different. I wish it were easier! Why did this happen to us?" I lamented.

"I don't know why infertility had to happen to you. We never really have all the answers. Why do some people have cancer? Why do others die in terrible accidents? I guess it is just how life goes. Infertility is your lot in life. It just wasn't meant to be. This is your cross to bear. Maybe you weren't meant to have children. We'll never know why. You should be grateful for what you do have."

This response was surprising and instantly made me shrink down deep inside myself. It hurt more because my defenses were down and I had allowed myself to be vulnerable. I had not had time to guard my heart or prepare for the pain.

The exchange continued, and the lump in the back of my throat grew as I stared silently at my hands, folded in my lap.

"You know, I could die tomorrow and leave my wife and children all alone. We just never know what adversity we may have to endure in this life. It is best to make the most of it. Move on."

I sat in disbelief. Tears were streaming down my face by this point in the conversation. The hum of the restaurant, the waiters coming and going, and the meal in front of me all faded away and I was consumed with emotion. How could someone who loves me say something so hurtful and not realize the effect it would have on me?

I was hurt, but I was also angry.

I mumbled an excuse and left for the sanctuary of the ladies' room without finishing my meal. This exchange minimized my infertility and my resulting emotional turmoil. Shock at the lack of empathy afforded to me and my all-encompassing grief kept me silent, locking my truth deep down to bear in secret. I would lie awake at night and think of the many things I wish I would have said in the restaurant that evening:

I could die tomorrow too, but maybe I won't. Perhaps you won't either, and you will live a long and happy life with your wife and your beautiful, healthy children. Maybe you will live the kind of life that allows you to watch your children grow up as you cherish the memories that come from a lifetime of health and happiness. Either way, I am going to have a great life too—even if it isn't the life I imagined.

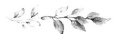

Throughout my years of infertility, when someone would make an insensitive comment, I became flustered, mumbled a response, and remained awkward and irrelevant for the remainder of our conversation. I found that if I talked about my infertility, it made everyone uncomfortable and usually led to quick changes of conversation. Eventually, Hoyt and I crafted a few standard replies to combat insensitive comments or when the usual question about how many children we have is asked.

With time, I learned that when an acquaintance makes an insensitive comment, I can either respond honestly and that acquaintance may feel uncomfortable for a second or two, or I can say nothing, regret staying quiet, hold onto that insensitivity and allow it to hurt my heart long past our initial interaction.

So, now, after seven years of questions and comments, I am honest. I say things like "I cannot have children," "I had a hysterectomy," or "I did not choose to be childless."

When someone advises me to adopt, I ask them if they'd recommend private, domestic, or international adoption, if they realize that adoption can cost up to $70,000, or if they had considered adopting instead of having biological children. When someone complains about their children or a woman who is "pregnant again" (insert incredulous eye roll), I talk about what a blessing a child is and how lucky that mother truly is to be pregnant.

I experienced one of the most empowering conversations in my healing process one afternoon with Dixie's husband, Danny. We were visiting for a few days at the lake. The campsite was quiet in the late afternoon glow of a perfect summer day. Dixie had been called in to work and our niece and nephew were playing contentedly. Hoyt, Danny and I were alone. In a quiet moment, Danny asked us, "So how are you doing—*really?*" This simple question instantly brought tears to my eyes—partly because my grief and sadness was still so fresh and raw and partly because no one had asked me how I was *really* doing.

With this simple question, Danny acknowledged my pain and my sorrow. He gave me the space to speak honestly. He offered no pity or advice. He wasn't alarmed or uncomfortable when my tears flowed freely. Instead, he listened quietly and let Hoyt and I talk about our hurt and our healing. At the end of the conversation, I felt connected, valued, and heard. My infertility was no longer my unspoken secret sorrow.

Chapter 31

When I received my initial diagnosis of uterine fibroids and endometriosis, I assumed that my condition would obviously directly affect my fertility—my reproductive system. After living with my diagnosis, I know now that infertility affects so much more. It touched all aspects of my health and wellbeing including my marriage, my finances, and my mental, emotional, and physical health. My friendships and family relationships were not immune either.

During the years of my fertility treatments, I put my life on hold because I was always waiting—for something. I waited for the right time, for after the next round of IVF, for weight loss, for the next surgery, for my body to heal, for my embryos to take hold. My waiting spilled over into all the areas of my life and colored the decisions I made—big and small.

Early on, when I still took for granted that one day soon I would become a mother, I designated one of our spare bedrooms to become our nursery. The walls in the bedroom were light grey, textured wallboard—a blank canvas. For seven years, I refused to paint that bedroom because I was waiting to design and decorate the space, transforming it into our nursery.

The room sadly sat empty and colorless. I kept the door firmly shut because the sight of the unoccupied room made my breath catch in my throat and tears instantly cloud my vision. This space symbolized all that I had dreamed of and lost. It was a cruel reminder that my babies were not here on earth with me. I felt cheated and angry. I was reminded that I was missing out on the joy of motherhood every time I opened the door. The room was strictly off limits.

Family photos have always been an important yearly tradition in my family. Growing up with a parent who was terminally ill instilled the importance of capturing moments and memories. Hoyt and I had photos taken early in our marriage but once my infertility took hold of our lives, neither Hoyt nor I had the desire to recall that particular period.

Shortly after we were married, my mom gave us a large, collage-style picture frame that we hung in our living room. It sat ready and waiting to be filled with beautiful, smiling pictures of Hoyt and me with our growing family. For seven years, the photo frame hung in our living room with stock photos of two expressionless Victorian-era girls in each of the frames. I was waiting for family photos of us with our newborn babies to fill these spaces. Those pictures wouldn't be coming, yet I couldn't bring myself to add any others. No one's photo would be important enough to earn a spot in that frame.

Hoyt and I were married when we were twenty-seven years old—an age when our friends and siblings started having their children in rapid succession. Hoyt and I would watch from our baby rollercoaster, wondering when it would be our turn to exit our wild ride and join our family and friends in parenthood. As one well-meaning family after another finished having their babies, they would bring me boxes and bags of baby supplies—bottles, crib sheets, adorable outfits, tiny shoes—and maternity clothes.

For years, I kept giant cardboard boxes of hand-me-down baby things and maternity clothes in the back of my closet in preparation for my growing belly. I looked at those big brown boxes every morning while I dressed, wishing that I could be choosing from inside its contents instead of from the items hung in my closet. I clung to the items in those boxes, wistfully imagining that one day soon I would know the wonder of motherhood. I tortured myself. I kept holding out hope that my "one day" would come. My life was on hold. I was caught in a loop and I couldn't break free.

As I shifted my life to embrace my post-hysterectomy childlessness, I started taking small, consistent steps to change my energy and my mindset. I painted my front and back doors a deep and elegant purple because the color makes me happy. I took down the awful, brown drapes that had hung in our living room since before we were married and replaced them with sheer white curtains that let the light into our home. No more darkness, only light.

I packed up all the maternity clothing and baby-related items stored in my closet and dropped them at a thrift shop with hopes that they would find their way to the women and children who need them. Donating these unused items made room in my closet for clothing that made me feel vibrant, beautiful, and confident.

A coat of soft, lilac-colored paint transformed the room that would've been our nursery into my writing room. I filled the space with stylish furniture and meaningful artwork. This room, which once held the painful reminder of our broken dreams, now makes me feel peaceful and inspired—it's a place just for me.

The quilting fabrics that my mom had purchased and prepared to turn into a beautiful baby blanket sat cut and ready at the bottom of her dresser drawer for years. This project—that had once held so much promise and excitement—was too painful for either Mom or I to quilt once childlessness became my reality. I had the beautiful blue and coral colored quilt finished by a local quilter instead. When it was done, I donated it to a woman's shelter. May it bring comfort, warmth, and security to a new mother and her bundle of joy.

Finally, I commissioned a dear friend to capture photos of Hoyt and I in our pasture—one of my favorite places on earth. The pasture is peaceful, serene, and has an incredible view. It is the perfect place to sit quietly, look out over the valley below, and plan for the future. The resulting photos are mounted in my collage frame and proudly displayed in our living room.

I started to do the things that made me happy. I did things that made me feel good. I lightened up my life, made my surroundings beautiful and meaningful. I considered what I wanted to bring forward into the future with me and I let everything else fall away. I made it my priority to do the things that are good for my soul and to say no to the things that don't bring me joy.

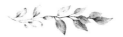

There is freedom in this little word: *no*. There are events to which I have learned to say no, all in the name of self-preservation. I still avoid attending most baby showers and first birthday parties. I find the baby-ogling, the birth stories, the parenting advice, and the questions of when it will be my turn, difficult.

I politely decline with a standard response that I have memorized and hangs on the tip of my tongue. I am always honest about my reasons for not attending. Sometimes I suggest a quiet cup of coffee where I can meet the new mom and baby, just us. I find it easier to express my joy for the new little one that way. Other times, I send a card with cash or ask my sister to deliver a gift and my well-wishes. I am always honest with myself and with the hostess. Being honest is easier than attending a shower when I'm not ready emotionally.

Hoyt and I tend to say, "No thank you," when invited to gatherings that are going to include large numbers of children—we find these sorts of events difficult. When a big group of parents with young children gather together for an event, the children tend to take over the day and the parents are consumed wholly by caring for their children (as it should be). Hoyt and I generally sit awkwardly together on the sidelines, watching the chaos unfold around us. We feel as though we can't relate. We tire of politely responding to story after story of children and babies and hockey practices and minivans.

These endless conversations leave me feeling as though my achievements and interests pale in comparison to motherhood. I return home feeling less—less of a woman, less interesting, less valuable. We are at a different point, in a different reality than other couples our age. This reality can feel isolating at times. Hoyt and I agreed that continuing these relationships was important but with boundaries that protect our emotional wellbeing. We also agreed to find friends with whom we could genuinely connect. We needed to find our people—friends who understand us, where we are, and where we've been. Here, we are free to be our childless selves.

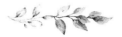

If I am honest with myself, I would admit the day I walked out of Dr. Mustache's office that very first time, I knew deep down I would not ever have children. My grieving process started all those years ago. While my conscious mind may have been researching fertility treatments and planning for babies, my subconscious mind was grieving what, deep down, I already knew.

For Hoyt, this was very different. He did not have seven years to grieve and to work through the stages of accepting this reality. Hoyt never entertained the thought that our fertility treatments would fail. Instead, he was the eternal optimist, sure everything would work out in our favor. For Hoyt, the death of our babies came as a devastating shock. Throughout this journey, I have often forgotten that infertility did not just happen to me. It happened to my husband, too.

Hoyt walked a different path than I did to come through our infertility. While some of the way we walked together, some parts we each had to go through alone. Many days the loss of our twins and our resulting childlessness threatened to tear us apart, pushing us further and further from each other and the love we share.

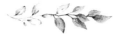

A successful marriage takes effort at the best of times and infertility put an extra strain on our relationship. Infertility influenced every decision, every moment, every experience we shared. I wish we could've taken time to do things together that gave us a chance to breathe, to do something fun, to have a break. I longed to feel carefree and happy again—the way I had early on in our relationship. Hoyt and I needed to remember the way we lit up around each other before the stress of infertility overshadowed our lives.

Choosing to embrace childlessness allowed us the opportunity for freedom and peace once again. I bought new, lacy underwear. I went out of my way to do kind or unexpected acts for Hoyt. We had sex spontaneously and to celebrate our love for each other, not because my ovulation predictor said we should.

Redefining our life together was a slow process that took hard work. We had to allow each other the time and space to feel how we each needed to feel and to grieve—even if our healing processes looked differently or ran on different schedules. We had to find a way to see outside of our own pain and to be strong for each other. We learned to be gentle with each other's souls. I needed Hoyt beside me through the muck and the mire that was my grief. He needed me, too—even if he was too tough to admit it.

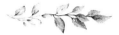

I love carbs (the more, the better). I am guilty of emotional eating and I hate exercising. That's the recipe for an unhealthy body. Shortly after my hysterectomy, Rhonda, after much prodding, discussing, and convincing, finally persuaded me to get serious about my physical self, my nutrition, and my health. I had a new appreciation for my body after my narrow escape from the dreaded colostomy bag and was finally ready to make some serious and lasting changes. I committed to putting myself first. I dedicated time each day to moving my body, eating exactly the foods my body needed at precisely the right times, and reading inspiring books to care for my spirit.

At first, it was hard. It was painful. Some days I couldn't sit down because I was so stiff and sore. Every day, I battled with myself as I worked through various excuses as to why I couldn't do my daily workout. It was hard—just as I expected.

What I didn't expect was how wonderful I started to feel. It was exhilarating to do something new, to stay committed to my health for more than a day or two, to feel my body moving, the see the strength of my muscles, and to realize the resilience of my spirit.

I became stronger. I found myself saying no to foods I had previously loved. My tastes changed. Suddenly, my familiar, favorite comfort foods tasted too sweet or too salty. I hated how bloated and tired I felt when I ate unhealthy foods. I focused on my nutrition and kept waking up every morning to spend time with myself—moving my body, meditating, and appreciating the miracle that was my body.

It was wonderful.

I started noticing differences in my body. I started seeing muscles where I didn't know my body had muscles. Inches started shrinking away and with them went wisps of the gloomy grey cloud that had hung over my head for so many years. Movement was a vital component of my healing.

With my commitment to my health and wellness, my life started to shift. It happened slowly at first, but soon I noticed changes. I discovered things I love to do. I gained confidence. I started reconnecting with friends and family whom I had distanced myself during my infertility. I thought about my future and made plans for the kind of life that held meaning and purpose for me—regardless of how society defined a meaningful life.

Despite its imperfections and inability to bear children, I was learning to love and appreciate my body. With each new physical challenge and each new level of my wellness, my appreciation grew. My lungs could breathe deeply. My legs were strong and carried me through my day. My heart beat out a rhythm in my chest. My digestive system was intact and fully functioning. I was free of pain. Gratitude seeped through my soul. I was alive. I was healthy. I was healing.

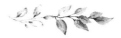

As I healed my soul, I was inspired to write a book to share the highs and lows of my baby rollercoaster. The inspiration would come and I would give myself a thousand reasons why I could never write a book. Then the feeling would go away...for a while. However, that sense of creative purpose always found its way back to me so one day, I told Hoyt, "I think I want to write a book, but I don't know how."

Hoyt is a black and white thinker—logical and rational. He reasoned, "Well if you want to write a book, it's very simple. Find a piece of paper and a good pen. Then, just write down what you want to say."

After some serious eye rolling, I did precisely that. I sat down at the computer and I wrote. As I started typing, my story started pouring out of my heart and onto the computer screen. As the words began to take shape in the form of sentences and paragraphs on the screen before me, the ache in my throat and the pain in my chest subsided. Since I had written my story and it was saved in the vast memory of my laptop, I no longer had to hold the pain and grief all in my heart. I could rest because I knew my journey was right there, written down, close to me if I needed it, but I didn't have to cling onto it so tightly.

I found relief and solace in my writing. It started as a therapeutic act for my soul, but it soon turned into something more. As I wrote hard and clear about what hurt me most, I realized I had an opportunity to reach out to other women around me who might be bearing their infertility in private, all alone, just as I had for so many years.

Chapter 32

I finally pushed the emergency stop button on my baby rollercoaster—for good this time. As my coaster car slowed and finally rolled to a stop, I lifted the safety bar, grabbed Hoyt's hand and together, we wobbled toward the exit gate of infertility, just the two of us. The rollercoaster came to life with a hum and left the gate to continue on for the rest of the couples aboard. Hoyt and I watched wistfully from the ground below.

Half glad to be on solid ground again and half broken-hearted to cut our ride short. Our wild ride left us dizzy, nauseated, and firmly resolved to enjoy the rest of our time together but without the adrenaline rush and thrill of any more amusement park rides.

In the sunset of our day at the fair, we quietly watch other couples and young families enjoying the rides and the amusements. We observe mothers lovingly wiping their toddler's sticky hands and faces. We see fathers protectively lathering goopy sunscreen onto their children's outstretched arms. We hear the excited shouts and laughter of families making memories to last a lifetime. The unconditional love that these parents have for their children is electric in the air.

We feel it.

We turn and walk into the sunset glow—hand in hand—knowing that while our baby rollercoaster wasn't what we dreamed it would be, the rest of the fair is pretty amazing too. We can make beautiful memories as a family of two. Our version of the amusement park is less sticky and sunburned, but pretty great just the same.

My heart, my marriage, and my bank account couldn't take another ride on infertility's unpleasant rollercoaster. I always thought that if childlessness really was a reality for my life that I would be comforted knowing I had exhausted every avenue (no matter the cost), tried every treatment (no matter how painful), and made my best attempt to adopt (no matter how invasive the process). But the truth is that I didn't feel better. I felt more depleted, more desperate, more devastated, and more in debt with every failed attempt to build our family.

My mental and emotional health suffered with each failed cycle as did my relationship with Hoyt. My turbulent ride through infertility left me with a skewed vision of my value as a woman and as a wife. It became obvious that it was time for us to leave the rollercoaster of emotions that accompanied our fertility treatments.

This is my story. My journey through the highs and lows of infertility and out the other side, to a great life. I wish I could write about our fabulous happily ever after, to tell you we persevered and tried one more time and it worked, or that we adopted and had a happy ending to our infertility story—but that was not to be the case for us. While this might not be how Hoyt and I envisioned our ride to end, we chose to walk away from building our family to chase after happiness on our own terms.

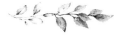

In my darkest nights, I remember being extremely angry with God or the Universe or Fate or whatever is out there yelling, "Fine then! If I can't have a baby, WHAT is my purpose here on Earth?!" I've asked that question over and over, partly scared of what the answer might be, but entirely ready to feel purpose and fulfillment in my life. The Universe gently nudged me and eventually shoved me in the direction of what I believe to be my purpose beyond motherhood.

I was blessed to have strong women in my life who surrounded me and encouraged me to reach for more. I applied for an administrative position and became Vice Principal of an elementary school.

I have always advocated for, taught, and loved other women's babies. This new role allows me to make change, to advocate harder, and to support women, children, and families in a whole new way. If I can't have my own babies, then maybe, just maybe, my purpose is to love and guide other women's children instead. My heart, my passion, and my purpose lie here.

Once I shook off the nausea and dizziness of my baby rollercoaster ride, I was able to open myself up to the endless possibilities available to me. There is this big, beautiful life waiting there for me to grab hold of, even though it might not be the life I imagined I would live. Your big, beautiful life is waiting for you, too.

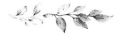

My boys will always hold a place in my heart, even if I can't hold them here on earth. Hoyt and I love our boys. We have dreamed of our boys and have longed for them since the day we met in his mother's back yard. We have yearned to see two tiny hearts beating in rhythm on an ultrasound screen. We have ached to hear our boys' first cries and to hold them warm and safe against our hearts where nothing bad could ever happen. We planned all the things we would teach our boys—how to run a ranch, how to always be kind even when it is hard, and how to love family with all their might.

Our sweet boys would've had a fabulous childhood full of tractor rides, baby calves, cookies fresh from the oven, and bedtime stories. These Colven brothers would have taken their place in the long line of proud prairie men in our family to assume ownership of the farm and to keep the legacy alive for another generation. Our boys would be smart and handsome, just like their dad, with golden blond hair and green eyes mischievously sparkling in the summer sunshine.

I would've loved to wash endless piles of dirty laundry, cook favorite meals, and fix countless ripped knees in jeans. I would've rocked our boys to sleep every night when they were babies. I would've watched every hockey game they played, even though I don't know a thing about hockey. First days at school, first trucks and first loves—I have imagined each milestone our boys would have passed. I will always wonder about the men that these boys would have grown up to be and I'm sad that I will never truly know—I can only imagine who they would've been. What I do know is no matter who our boys were meant to become, I would have been standing proudly by their side every step of the way to love them and support them and guide them as only a mother can.

I'll always cherish the days I was privileged to hold our boys in my womb, the days I was able to shelter my babies and nourish them and protect them, the days they were mine. For now, I'll treasure those memories until I can hold my boys in my arms one day when I get to Heaven. Until then, I will keep my sweet boys tucked away in the place in my heart that I have saved just for them. My heart will never forget my baby rollercoaster ride or my boys—the experience has changed me forever.

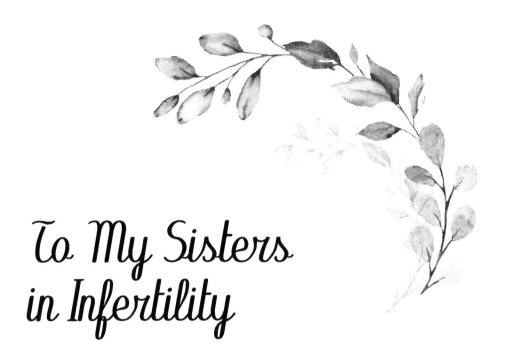

To My Sisters in Infertility

You are reading these words because you, too, have experienced loss or infertility. I may not know you personally, but I know you. I know you because I am you. I see you. I understand you. I feel what you feel. I have cried your tears. I have been where you are. I have felt the pain—both physical and emotional. I have battled demons. I have whispered my fears in the dark. I have cried until my pillow was soaked and my eyes were too swollen to open.

When you have another negative pregnancy test, know I have been there on the bathroom floor in tears, too. When you find yourself alone at a baby shower, know I have also felt your secret pain. When you read another pregnancy announcement and dream of yours, know that I understand that undeniable ache in your heart. When you find yourself at the fertility clinic to try just one more time, know I have sat in that seat, too. When you slowly lose more and more of your hope for the life you thought you'd have, know I have experienced that loss, too. When you once again rebuild and redefine your life, know that I have been resilient, too.

You are not alone.

You are beautiful and strong and you've done everything right. You are not broken. Infertility is not your fault. I understand the pain and disappointment you feel in the depths of your soul. But I also know that the pain will not last forever. Infertility will change you, but it doesn't have to define you or break you. You have the power and strength inside of you to heal your soul.

There are many ways to build a family if you choose—but I also know that a family of two is still a family. You can exit your baby rollercoaster and go on to find your purpose in this life—beyond motherhood. With time, fulfillment and joy will overcome your sorrow. I know this because I have been where you are.

Take comfort in my story. Take strength from my journey. Find hope in my words. Know that this is not the end for you. You will find your way through your grief. You will be happy once again. The ache in your chest will subside and your tears will come less frequently. New ideas and opportunities will present themselves. Eventually, a subtle shift in your hopes and dreams will occur and space will open up for you to explore your creativity and strengths.

You will live a great big, beautiful life. Yes, it will be different than you imagined, and yes, it might be different than it's supposed to be. Yes, you will have to work harder than you thought possible, but it will be your life, created just for you. Confidently step off your baby rollercoaster and step into the rest of your life. I promise it will be worth it.

Be brave. Keep going. Breathe.

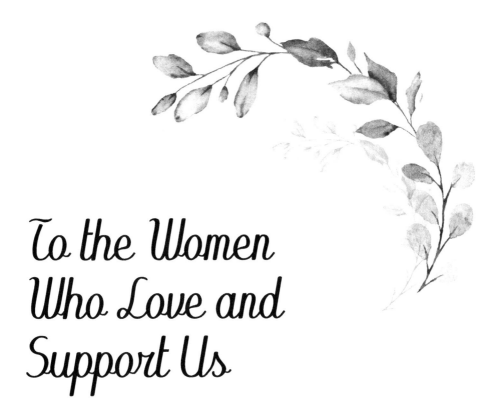

To the Women Who Love and Support Us

Showing your support for a childless woman or a couple working through infertility requires you to pause and reflect on the language you use, the assumptions you make, and the sorts of questions you ask. Choose your words carefully and avoid these common questions and statements:

- Do you have children? How many children do you have?
- Didn't you want to have children?
- Don't wait too long.
- Your time will come.
- Your clock is ticking.
- Did you try _____?
- My friend used this herbal tea/detox/diet/healing crystals and it cured her infertility. She is pregnant right now.

- Stop trying and it'll happen. Relax and it'll happen. Go on vacation and it'll happen. Be patient and it'll happen.
- Did you hear that _____ is pregnant again? She wasn't even trying.
- Maybe it wasn't meant to be. God has other plans for you. It wasn't part of God's plan. This is your lot in life.
- Everything happens for a reason.
- You'll see your babies in heaven.
- You can try again.
- Maybe the next cycle will be successful.
- My friend/cousin/neighbor also had endometriosis and she has four kids.
- You can take my kids.
- Enjoy your freedom.
- Babysitting is a great form of birth control.
- What about adoption? You could always adopt. Why don't you adopt? I know someone who adopted from Africa/the province/the Ukraine/Florida.
- You are a mother to many—you are a teacher.
- You can spend time with your nieces and nephews instead.
- You can be a "special" auntie.
- Children are so expensive. You are lucky, you must have lots of money.
- My morning sickness/swollen ankles/weight gain is just awful.
- You're so lucky you can sleep in/travel/have nice furniture.
- You wouldn't understand, you're not a mom/grandma.
- I didn't know true love until I became a mother/grandmother.
- Being a mother/grandmother is the best job in the world.
- Giving birth is the most powerful act a woman can do.

As an alternative to asking if a woman has children, consider other ways to begin a casual conversation.

- What are you passionate about right now?
- What are you working on at the moment?
- Have you travelled anywhere exciting recently?
- Have you tried this new restaurant?
- What are you reading?
- Tell me about your family.

Questions such as this allow for deeper answers, more connection, and more freedom to express our true selves. These subtle shifts in conversation matter. They allow a childless woman to leave the exchange feeling valued and heard.

For deeper conversations, ask open-ended questions like:

- How are you doing—really?
- What's the hardest part of your infertility?
- What are you most afraid of in your treatment/ appointment/test/childlessness?
- What do you wish that the people closest to you could understand?
- How can I support you in this moment?
- What do you need right now?

It means a lot to know that you care enough to take the time to ask me how I'm really doing and to understand more of my childlessness.

Holidays and Celebrations

Celebrate the childless women in your life. Go to dinner at the best restaurant in town when she applies to begin her Master's degree. Send flowers when she is promoted at work. Attend her puppy's extravagant first birthday party and don't forget to bring a gift. Applaud her home renovation. Rejoice when she finishes her quilt, completes her masterpiece, hires a publisher, or makes her best time yet in a race. Seemingly small moments and milestones are incredibly important in our childless lives. We need you there beside us, celebrating our achievements and special events—even though they look differently than yours.

Holidays are hard. As a childless woman, I feel pressure that seasons and holidays need to "look" a certain way. Back to School, Christmas, Mother's Day, birthdays—these important events are woven into our culture. These seasons and special days are what bring joy to our lives and create memories. But what does Christmas morning look like when you don't have excited children running to sit under the sparkling lights of the tree, eyes dancing, as they squeal with delight over the gift that Santa has delivered?

Hoyt and I had to redefine what the Christmas season meant for us. We needed time to find our own traditions—just the two of us. Some years we chose to spend Christmas with our families and other years, we chose to be at home, celebrating quietly together.

Invite and include the childless woman in your circle. Allow her the opportunity to decide if she'd like to attend your holiday party or Mother's Day brunch. Don't feel offended if she politely declines your offer. Allow your childless friend or family member to host holiday meals if they choose. Don't expect that they will always travel to you because they don't have children and it is "easier" for them.

Find simple ways to be supportive through special seasons and holidays. Send a "Best Auntie in the World" mug or a basket of goodies on Mother's Day. Go out of your way to make birthdays memorable. Call during the Christmas season to check in with the childless woman in your life. Remember that we won't be posting back to school photos of our adorable children in September. Be sensitive to the reality that these holidays and special occasions—while happy and exciting for you—can trigger grief and sadness for us. Connection is the antidote to the separation that exists when a woman compares her childless life to that of her fertile friends and family. One way to create connection is to be present and to start a conversation.

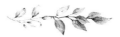

Most of all, love us through whatever comes—the highs and lows, the uncertainty, the hormones, the mood swings, the grief, the hope. No matter the outcome, we need you there beside us for when the dust settles and we need to put the pieces of our lives back together. The trauma of infertility will linger long past a failed cycle. The trauma will even persist if a woman is blessed with a child. Infertility changes you. It becomes part of who you are and how you see the world. Remember this and have empathy for those who have lived with infertility.

Resources

These women have inspired and comforted me throughout my healing after the unspoken secret sorrow of my infertility. May you also find inspiration and comfort through their words, their example, and connection with women who also know the sorrow of infertility.

Girl, Wash Your Face
By Rachel Hollis

In this book, Rachel Hollis reminded me that I am in control and have the power to create the life I want. She inspired me to keep promises to myself and to set new and exciting goals.

The Universe Has Your Back
By Gabrielle Bernstein

In this book, Gabrielle Bernstein's words gave me strength when I was down and inspired me to look for joy when I was experiencing deep emotional pain. The awareness that the Universe was supporting me, even in my grief, was a great source of comfort.

The Gifts of Imperfection
By Brené Brown

In this book, Brené Brown showed me how to embrace and accept all of myself, including my childlessness. I learned to stop chasing after the image of the life I thought I should have and to live authentically.

Heavy Flow: Breaking the Curse of Menstruation
By Amanda Laird

In this book, Amanda Laird taught me about the history of period shame and stigma. She gave me a unique perspective regarding menstruation as well as other topics related to women's health and wellness. This is a "must-read" for women everywhere.

Online Resources

Joining online groups and communities has allowed me to connect with other women who share similar experiences and stories. Here, I am free to be myself and to share my infertility. Here, I am able to see that there is life after infertility. Connection with these women has truly helped to heal my soul.

Facebook Groups

Search Facebook for an online infertility group in your area. You may also consider searching for a group specific to your condition, such as endometriosis.

Instagram Communities

Search using appropriate hashtags on Instagram to find and connect with other women who share similar experiences. Some hashtags to consider include: #childlessnotbychoice, #endometriosisawareness, #hysterectomy, #infertilityawareness, #lifeafterinfertility.

Beachbody Fitness Groups

Beachbody on Demand is a fitness and nutrition streaming service that I invested in after healing from my hysterectomy. These at-home workout programs helped me to take control of my physical health. Daily exercise supported my mental health. The online fitness groups connected me with other women who shared similar health and wellness goals which motivated me to keep working toward my own goals. Follow me on Instagram @janice_colven for information on my monthly challenge groups.

Acknowledgments

Countless people have supported, empowered, and inspired me throughout the process of sharing my truth in the words on these pages. I thank you and send you each love and many blessings.

To my husband, Hoyt. You inspired me to have the courage to write this book and to share our story. You stood strong beside me through the trauma of infertility. Thank you.

To my sister, Rhonda. You are my angel. You will never know how much your selfless act of love meant to me. Gratitude wells up in my soul each time I think of our embryos or of you. Thank you for sharing the burden of my sorrow and for showing me how to follow my heart.

To my brother-in-law, Kyle. You are kind and generous beyond measure. You made me smile and laugh on some of the hardest days I have ever endured. Thank you.

To my mom, Joan. You have loved me through the darkest days of my life as only a mother can. You have shown me strength and resilience that I can only hope to emulate. Thank you, Mom.

To my mother-in-law, Darlene. You introduced me to the love of my life. For that, I am grateful. You had empathy for the pain of our loss and loved Hoyt and me both through our grief. Thank you.

To my sister-in-law, Dixie. You were there, always. Thank you.

To my friend, Angela. You told your story and you listened to mine. You offered connection and empathy during a time when I desperately needed both. I am so blessed to have you in my life.

To my publisher, Jeanne. You helped me to take this book from good—to great. You believed that together, we could make a difference in the lives of women. Thank you for making me an author.